Health according to the Scriptures

Experience the Joy of Health according to Our Creator

I say these things so that you might be saved.
—John 5:34

Paul Nison

©2010 Paul Nison

All Rights Reserved. No part of this book may be reproduced by any means, except for brief quotations embodied in articles and reviews, without the express written consent from the author.

Disclaimer

This book is not intended as medical advice. When going on a natural diet, there is always some risk involved. Because of this, the author, publisher, and/or distributors of this book are not responsible for any adverse detoxification effects or consequences resulting from the use of any suggestions or procedures described herein.

Printed in Canada

Fourth Edition, January 2010
Third Edition, August 2007
Second Edition, May 2006
First Edition, September 2005

343 Publishing Company
P.O. Box 16156
West Palm Beach, FL 33416

www.paulnison.com
www.torahlifeministries.org

Editor: Bob Avery (bobavery@umich.edu)
Layout and Design: Kira A. Long
Cover: Enrique Candioti

ISBN # 978-0-9675286-4-9
Nutrition/Diet   Health   Religion

DEDICATION

This book is dedicated to the ancient Hebrew scribes who retained our great Creator's names in their original Paleo-Hebrew forms and lived according to the Torah.

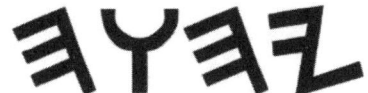

If you are sick or know someone who is sick, here is practical knowledge and truth from the Scriptures which will reveal how to avoid and cure sickness. This book is for you!

WARNING! Once you read it, you can no longer use the excuse "I didn't know that." Then what will you do? Your health will depend on it!

> *So then, anyone who knows the right thing to do and fails to do it is committing a sin.* —James 4:17

Contents

What People Are Saying About This Book.. ix
Foreword by Jordan Rubin xi
Foreword by Pastor David Roberts xiii
Acknowledgments xv
Introduction xvii
Notes to the Reader xxvii

Part 1: My Commandments Are Not Burdensome
The Wise Shall Prosper   1

Chapter 1
From Disease to Wellness 3
Your Words Are Healing to All My Flesh

Chapter 2
Keeping Your Word 11
Commit Yourself to His Instructions

Chapter 3
Freedom 17
The Truth Shall Set You Free

Chapter 4
The Power of Adaptation 25
Let Yahweh Transform You into a New Person

Chapter 5
The Power of Temperance 33
Yahweh is Near to All Those Who Call Him

Chapter 6
The Scriptures: Use Them or Lose Them 37
The Teaching of His Word Gives Light

Chapter 7
Knowledge is Key: Listen and Obey 45
That Is the Duty of Every Believer

Part 2: Diet according to the Scriptures   51

Chapter 8
How We Have Forsaken Yahweh's Diet Plan 53
Let Each Generation Tell Its Children of Your Mighty Acts

Chapter 9
Nutrition according to the Scriptures 59
It Is Better to Trust in Yahweh than to Put Confidence in Man

Chapter 10
Yahweh's Designed Eating Plan 63
May Your Eye Take Delight in Following His Ways

Chapter 11
Yahweh Said Don't Touch That 73
A Person without Self-Control Is Like a City with Broken-down Walls

Chapter 12
Yahweh's Approved Foods 95
He Gives Justice to the Oppressed and Food to the Hungry

Chapter 13
Beyond Diet: Supplements and Herbs 109
Life Is More than Just Bread Alone

Chapter 14
Misunderstood Scriptures about Food and Diet 111
The Wise Shall Understand

Part 3: Divine Design — Yahweh's Schedule   115

Chapter 15
How We Were Designed to Eat 117
Do Not Add to or Take Away from His Words on How to Eat

Chapter 16
When We Were Designed to Eat 131
There Is a Time for Every Purpose under the Sun

Chapter 17
Set Times to Eat 143
Yahweh Separated the Day from the Night for a Reason

Part 4: Whom Do You Worship?   **165**

Chapter 18
We Make an Idol Out of Our Food 167
No One Is Able to Serve Two Masters

Chapter 19
Meeting Your Emotional Needs 179
Yahweh Hears the Cries of the Righteous

Chapter 20
Dealing with People 181
Remove me Far from Vanity

Part 5: Healing according to the Scriptures   **189**

Chapter 21
Disease or No Disease 191
Choose Life and You Shall Live

Chapter 22
Healing according to the Scriptures 201
The Fear of Yahweh Leads to Life

Chapter 23
The Formula for Health 217
He Will Heal All Disease

Part 6: In the End It Will Be As It Was at the Beginning   **221**

Chapter 24
Putting a Plan Together 223
Seek the Kingdom of Yahweh above All Things

Chapter 25
Go in Good Health 231
Seek His will, and He Will Direct Your Path

Conclusion 237
List of Clean Meats and Unclean Meats 243
Recipes 245
Resources 255
About the Author 257
Suggested Reading 261
Prayers 263
Index 265
Torah Life Ministries 270
Order Form 272

What People Are Saying About This Book

This Book Is a Must Read!

Are you searching for better health? Then this is one book that is a must read. Paul Nison seeks to impart the balance between Scriptures, science, and the real world. He strikes a balance between Moses and Jesus, and that is not an easy task! In *Health according to the Scriptures*, Paul presents a balance between the often-misunderstood differences between the Old and New Covenants.

In *Health according to the Scriptures*, you will be challenged to rethink entrenched beliefs that have destroyed the health of believers and agnostics alike. The junk Western diet is not our friend. Science when divorced from the Scriptures is not our friend either. We must get back to the Creator's guidelines, back to health, body, soul, and spirit. As we integrate and wisely practice scriptural guidelines, the joyful opportunity to rescue the health of this generation becomes ours — as well as to rescue the health of our children and grandchildren. In fact, that challenge is actually one of our highest callings!

Therefore, I wholeheartedly recommend that you carefully and prayerfully dig into this groundbreaking book. Paul has done us a service by reminding us to get back to our foundations, back to the guidelines that undergird our creation. I can guarantee you will find more Scriptures on health in this book than you knew existed — carefully hidden, but now revealed in the pages of both the Old and New Covenants. Take a new look at the scriptural wisdom and guidelines presented. Your health might depend on it!

—**Dr. Roger L. DeHaan,** author of *We Don't Die, We Kill Ourselves!*; *Our Foods are Killing Us!*; and also *Restoring the Creation Mandate: Healing or People, Pets, Plants, & the Planet!*

Your Teachings Have Changed My Life!

I have just finished your new book. Great job! I wish there were some way to get a copy in front of every congregation leader in this country. So many of us in leadership need to realize that we must stop picking and choosing the parts of Torah we want to obey. We have a greater responsibility to address the hard issues. Lifestyle changes are a hard issue and provide active obedience to the Word. Your teachings have changed my life by opening my eyes to this area of Torah. Keep the faith and battle on.

—Pastor Earl Walters

I Recommend This Book

If you are ready to reclaim your health, to live a disease-free lifestyle, or to eat your way out of a prevailing illness, this book points you in the right direction. *Health according to the Scriptures* goes far beyond the rigors of a good diet; it's a spiritual awakening to the Father's will for our natural lives. A multiplicity of books have been written about diets and fads that have exploded on the scene of late. *Health according to the Scriptures* is neither a fad nor a diet. It's a commitment to improve one's overall existence while submitting to Yahweh's plan for healthy living. I recommend this book to everyone who's serious about living a healthy lifestyle according to the Scriptures. Be blessed as you discover what Yahweh is saying concerning His health plan for you and your family.

—Pastor Robert J. Brady, Kol Davar Beit Midrash

Foreword by Jordan Rubin

Each and every person was created by God to live a long and abundant life. The Bible, long thought of as merely a spiritual book, is what I believe to be God's plan for our well-being in body, soul, and spirit. God promises us extraordinary health if we follow His commandments (Exodus 15:26) and listen to His voice. Unfortunately, in today's fast-paced, technology-based society, we have broken nearly all of the age-old health principles outlined in God's Word, the Bible.

Paul Nison's *Health according to the Scriptures* is a valuable resource for anyone who seeks to know and understand God's plan for complete health and healing. I rejoice when an in-depth book on Bible-based health and wellness appears on the market, especially one from a friend like Paul. His own journey to health through the Scriptures will inspire many. His knowledge and understanding of God's Word will motivate even the most hesitant reader as he or she turns each page.

This book could not have been published at a more propitious time. With the increase of obesity, cardiac disease, diabetes, cancer, digestive disorders, and a host of other illnesses in our world, this book will prove to be a welcome inspiration for all who seek wholeness in body, soul, and spirit.

If you love to study God's Word as I do and you are looking for Bible-based answers to your health issues, you will enjoy the insights that Paul Nison offers. God never intended for us to be sick. It was His plan from the beginning that we lead vibrant, long, and healthy lives. Paul Nison unveils some scriptural truths and secrets that prove that God has a plan not only for our souls and spirits, but for our bodies as well.

I encourage you to put what Paul has written into practice. He has done us a profound service by illuminating the path to health through God's Word.

—Jordan Rubin, Founder and CEO of Garden of Life and author of New York Times best-seller *The Maker's Diet.*

Foreword by Pastor David Roberts

Health according to the Scriptures is a brilliant exposition, containing wonderful expressions of knowledge and enlightenment that explore the values of the true wealth of health. More importantly, this book will also help you establish the spiritual understanding of the created being that is called human. This book is a template of knowledge, insightfulness and wisdom — a creation produced by experiences in life that will benefit all who read it.

This book is filled with information on how to enjoy the abundance of life that Our Creator Yahweh has provided for those who obey Him and all His instructions. These instructions include His proper dietary laws. If followed, they will sustain us with "wealth and health" and give us the fullness of life that we all desire.

It is written from a poetic tapestry of experience and knowledge that gives us great erudition of the riches of The Most High One, Yahweh. The information is a great comprehension of the complexity of Yahweh's true designs for man to live life in a way that is not only healthy, but creates an environment of refreshing spirituality, with anticipation for today, an appreciation for the beauty of life, and a greater awareness of what will cause us to miss out on a healthy and productive lifestyle.

This knowledge gives us understanding so we can have great health in order to bring a true, invigorated worship to Yahweh our Creator. The sagaciousness of this book will serve as a paradigm for generations to come for a well-balanced life of robustness, creating an invigorating life and the discipline to sustain wellness in health and the healing process that begins in the inward parts (mind). This book will inspire and influence your actions to live a wonderful and healthy lifestyle.

A tremendous Inspiration comes from Scripture (Katuv):

> *Beloved, I wish above all things that you may prosper* [tsaw-lakh'] *and be in health* [mar-pay'], *even as your being prospers.*
> —3 John (Yochanan) 1:2

The value and importance of a vigorous mind, body, and spirit can happen if we allow the knowledge of this book to generate the wonders of a health-inspired lifestyle. A healthy lifestyle will produce a pleasant expression of our inward being that will be transmitted in the beauty of our smiles and facial expression, a brightness that can only be the expression of the wellness of a sound, wholesome, and well-balanced mind and body.

Health according to the Scriptures by Brother Paul Nison creates an oasis for us that will provide a refuge of relief from a lifestyle that tends to be filled with many handicaps of bad food choices that never energize us, to a lifestyle that is filled with a rebirth of a more purposeful life. Let the energies of life begin with this work of passion.

The book you have in your hand is a wellspring of healthy knowledge. Bless you, Brother Paul, and also your wife as well, who helps encourage you in this work. To you, Brother Paul, your wife, and all readers, I say to you, "Yev-arech-echah," Yahweh bless you.

—David Roberts, Pastor of Victory Community,
www.yahwehsword.org

Acknowledgments

First, I owe a very special thanks to my wife Andrea — the most beautiful woman in the world — a true blessing to my life.

In addition, I owe special thanks to—

- all my friends who have been praying for me through the years, far too many to name here. I'm so grateful for your help and friendship.

- all the members of my family, who have always been supportive, no matter how much they might not have fully agreed with my ideas.

- all the health educators I've interviewed or whose books I've read on the raw food diet and/or health improvement.

- Bob Avery for editing this edition of the book and Joel Brody for editing the original text.

- Enrique Candiotti for the beautiful cover design and Kira Long for the layout of the book.

- Jordan Rubin for his foreword, wisdom, and friendship.

- Dr. Fred Bisci, who has generously shared his wisdom, friendship, and prayers — ever available to give uplifting advice.

- Brother Doug Mitchell for his knowledge and permission to use his writings from his website about the correct daily eating schedule we should follow and also for permission to excerpt from the book *The Entering Wedge*, published by Victor T. Houteff for the Entering Wedge Society of America. You can see this book for free on the Internet at: http://www.thebranch.org/Bible_Vegetarianism_Food_Combinations_VT_Houteff.

- Dr. Roger DeHaan for his suggestions with this manuscript.

- Jordan Rubin for his foreword and passion to get this message out.

- my spiritual team: Baruch Bobo and Pastors Willard Cooper, Doug Mitchell, David Roberts, Allen Stanfield, and Earl Walters for all their knowledge, openness, and prayers.

- Yahweh's Congregation (www.yahwehsword.org) and Pastor David Roberts for his weekly inspiration and great preaching of the true message of Yeshua, as well as pamphlets that provided some of the text in the preface of this book.

- all my friends who welcomed me into their homes over the years. Your kindness was of great help — an ongoing inspiration I will never forget.

- and above all, to our Heavenly Father Yahweh, Hallelu-Yah!

Introduction

I take no pleasure in the death of wicked people. I only want them to turn from their wicked ways so they can live. —Ezekiel 33:11 [NLT]

When I was 20 years old, I was diagnosed with *inflammatory bowel disease*, a deadly disease medical doctors still have no cure for. Against my doctor's advice, I changed my diet and lifestyle and healed my condition at 22 years old. I was so thankful for my recovery that I wanted to find every tactic possible to help others tormented with health challenges, especially those who seemed to have no hope in sight to restore their health. My own healing experience led me to believe people should never give up hope. My recovery convinced me that diet plays a huge role in causing and healing from disease. But I knew there was more than just diet alone. It was obvious that emotional issues and stress also had an extensive influence on the condition of my body.

One day, it was presented to me that there are spiritual issues that can result in physical disease. At the time, I was searching for a spiritual path to follow myself, not believing in one particular path. I figured if one god had countless solutions, various gods would have loads of answers.

It wasn't until years later when I was giving a lecture that this man I met afterwards informed me that the Bible was the greatest health book ever written. Up to that point, the only scripture I knew was Genesis 1:29 that declared man's food should be fruits and vegetables. I was all in favor of that scripture because the solution to my healing was eating a diet of only raw fruits, vegetables, nuts, and seeds. Beyond that verse, I had no intention to read the Scriptures. However, after he mentioned the Bible contained messages about health, I was curious to find out if what he was declaring was accurate.

I was very interested to know why he thought the Bible was a better health book than my book that took me years to write. I had tons of information about all aspects of health. Up to that point, I'd read or seen many health books and articles on health. I was sure there might have been some books out there that were just as good and maybe better, but I didn't see any at that time that had the wisdom I was sharing in my book and lectures. I didn't want to seem like I knew it all, but after being on the brink of death with a deadly disease that doctors had no cure for, I felt I had more answers than the occasional doctor who wrote a book, or even a best-selling author at that time. I believed this because none of them were as sick as I was, and none of them understood how to heal disease the way I did. So I looked at this fellow and I said I'd like to see the book.

His reply was simply, "Okay, but you have to make me a promise before I give you the book."

This piqued my interest even more. "Here's the deal," he said, "I will give you the book for free, and if you don't find it to be the best book ever written on the topic of health, give it back to me; but if you do agree with me that it is the best health book ever written, you have to tell other people about it."

Of course I agreed to his deal. Just when he was about to give me the book, he told me one more part of the deal: before letting him know what I thought about it, I had to promise I would read the whole book cover to cover in order. No problem, sir, now can I have the book? He handed it to me. I looked at the cover, and it said, *The Scriptures*.

Normally I would have told him I wasn't a religious person and given him the book back as I did many times before when someone handed me the Scriptures. But this time was different; I was excited to read the book and prove him wrong. I wanted him to see that it could not possibly have more information about health than my book.

After reading the whole book, I can say I was very wrong, and I haven't given him the book back. So, because I am a man of my word, now I have to tell everyone else about it.

The Scriptures are truly the best health book ever written. They are about complete health from a physical, emotional, and spiritual standpoint. If anyone disagrees, I make that same deal that fellow made with me. If you don't agree, fine, but read the whole book in order before developing an opinion.

If you want to identify the supreme way to eat for ultimate health, search the Scriptures, and you will locate your answer. The Scriptures (James 1:17) proclaim all that is good comes from Yahweh (Our Creator, commonly referred to as, God, Lord, Adonai). It is a waste of time searching for someone or something that understands more than our own Maker about the human body and how to keep it functioning at its best. Our Creator is the finest doctor, healer, and supplier. Everything we need comes from Him.

The health puzzle facing so many of us today can be solved with simple scriptural answers:

The keys to good health are

1. Learn what Yahweh wants for you, and pray about it!
2. Take action, and live according to His instructions!
3. Enjoy all His blessings!

This exciting discovery means we all have the capability to be healthy!

Everything and everyone has a purpose in life, including us. To carry out that purpose, we must be healthy. Yahweh made our bodies so amazingly to overcome disease and discomfort. Now we must visit what the Scriptures say about health and healing to get back our good health that Yahweh promised us. It is my prayer that this book will help you accomplish that.

The reason I was led to write this book was because as I started teaching in churches, I noticed to my surprise more prayer for the healing of disease than for any other topic. I wondered how these people had the greatest health book ever written in their hands and were still experiencing disease. I thought that instead of praying for healing of disease, they should have been praising Yahweh for wonderful health. I was mystified.

After more time in various assemblies and churches, I became aware of the problem. The majority of people weren't reading their Scriptures, and the people who were, weren't following the instructions.

The first thought bewildered me. How can people not be inspired to read the instruction book of life, Our Creator's very own guidelines on how to live a long life in health, peace, and joy? After realizing it had taken me many years also to open the book and read it for the first time, I understood the answer. Each of us has to be ready to explore the information firsthand for ourselves. Often it takes a dramatic near-death experience for someone to be ready to see what our Creator has to offer.

The second thought revealed a more common issue, people reading but not willing to follow what the Scriptures say. Whether it is because lack of faith, lack of understanding, deception, or addiction to living certain lifestyles, many so-called believers today are not willing to entirely change their lives to go along with the instructions of the Scriptures, found in the Torah.

The sad fact is that we live in a world today where the majority of people have little interest in learning and obeying Yahweh's Word. We have more people living today against the guidelines found in the instruction book of life than ever before. We are also in a time when there is more disease and sickness than ever before. It doesn't take a genius to figure out the connection.

The closer our relationship is with Yahweh, the more we will identify and understand what He desires for us. He does not want us to be sick, and He never wanted us to suffer with disease. He wants us to love Him and understand that He created us, and He can keep us healthy.

> *Yahweh ordered us to observe all these laws, to fear Yahweh our Creator, always for our own good, so that He might keep us alive, as we are today.*
>
> *It will be righteousness for us if we are careful to obey all these instructions before Yahweh our Creator, just as He ordered us to do.*
> —Deuteronomy 6:24-25

Deuteronomy 4:1 tells us we are to listen and obey, so we may live! All of Scripture has this same message. We are not instructed to do any more or any less than study, obey, and believe! Yahweh will take care of everything else, showering us with many blessings if we just do those three things.

If you want to live a long, healthy, joyful life, you need to realize that we are all going to die one day, and we can assure our eternal salvation only by the blood of our Messiah Yeshua (commonly called today Jesus). However, it's by keeping Torah (Yahweh's instructions and guidelines) that we are blessed with great health and joy while in our physical, earthly body.

In Deuteronomy 28, we are clearly shown the blessings and curses that coincide with obedience and disobedience. Disease is the result of sin. What is sin? Disobedience is sin! There are a few who may experience disease not as a result of sin, but for the glory of Yahweh. An example is the blind man in John 9. However, most people experience disease as a result of their lack of responsibility and lack of action for their own welfare.

It says in Scripture that many are called, but few are chosen (Matthew 22:14). However, I believe the correct translation is, "Many are called, but few choose." We each have a choice, and our actions reveal our hearts. If you seek to follow master Yahweh's plan, He will supply all your needs and bless you. You have to take responsibility for your choices. Many people do not like to confess it, but deep within their hearts, they realize the way they live and the choices they make result in the condition of their overall health or lack of it.

There are many good-hearted believers attending assemblies all over the world who are being deceived about the role of responsibility and obedience to Torah (the commandments, will, and guidelines of Yahweh). Consistent with the idea of grace without works, they experience the same diseases as nonbelievers.

It may be hard to comprehend my message because if what I am suggesting is accurate, everyone will be diagnosed with disease in one form or another because we all sin. Yahweh provided us with the magnificent gift of His Son, Yeshua, who shed His blood for us for those times we are not perfect. That is the distinction from all the other religions of this world. When you decide to follow Yahweh, you always have a savior. The blood of Yeshua will wash away those times when you are weak. However, that grace will not cleanse a disobedient heart. Grace is not a justification to keep living in sin. Grace is Yahweh's mercy to give you time to get stronger and closer with Him. Grace without works is dead, and works without Yeshua are nothing. We need both to be blessed!

If you have a firm understanding of the Word, it will be harder to be deceived. The Scriptures tell us many people are destroyed because of lack of knowledge (Hosea 4:6).

What do you do once you attain the knowledge? Knowledge is insignificant without action. In fact, the Scriptures say if you know something is good for you and do not do it, to you it is sin (James 4:17). If we never discovered what we were doing was harmful for us, there could be an excuse not to do it; however, once it is revealed that it is harmful, we no longer have the excuse that "I didn't know." The more we have been made aware of it, the more accountable we should be.

> *If I had not come and spoken to them, they wouldn't be guilty of sin; but now, they have no excuse for their sin.* —John 15:22

People may ask, "What if we didn't know?" That is more reason to study Scripture, so we can learn what is beneficial and what is of Yahweh.

> *"Whoever has ears to hear with, let him hear!"* —Luke 8:8

Yeshua came to reveal to man the will of His Father in heaven. For the Son of man was not sent to destroy souls, but to make them live (Ezekiel 33:11, Luke 9:56).

Whether you comprehend it or not, if you don't fully seek to obey His will for your life, your chances of getting disease will be immense! Yahweh is near to all those who choose to obey Him (James 4:8). The more we seek His path, the more He blesses us with wisdom and understanding. Disease is usually the result of us choosing to take our own path instead of the one He has laid out for us.

Deuteronomy 4:4 reveals to us that everyone who is faithful to Yahweh will survive (be saved). But it also shows us in Deuteronomy 9:14 that Yahweh will destroy everyone who seeks to follow other gods and the ways of man (by war, hunger, or *dis-*

ease). There is only one way to ensure we will endure: as Yeshua told us, Yahweh is the only way!

I have done my best to present the message in this book. My prayer is that you haven't overlooked this significant message I'm trying to convey to you about your health. What you eat is extremely critical, and this book will reveal to you the valuable message about eating according to the Scriptures. However, it is not only what goes in your mouth, but also what comes out of your heart that determines your health. If you live in obedience to Yahweh and *always* seek to honor and please Him, Yahweh will bless you with *every* kind of good fruit, and you will grow and learn more and more as you continue to draw closer to Yahweh (Colossians 1:10).

I see countless people in the health field searching for other ways to attain great health, but there is no other way in the history of the world that has the power that Yahweh has. History speaks for itself. Praise Yahweh that we can be with Him if we choose. No food, doctor, special diet, or exercise is going to give us the protection and blessings that He can give us.

I understand the urge to rely on numerous methods of healing. However, few of these are from Yahweh, and if you want to be healthy and enjoy our Creator's awesome power, you must detach from putting your faith in things that are not from Yahweh.

Deuteronomy 5:8-9 warns us that we must not have any idols in our lives or bow down and worship any other gods. If we do these things, not only will we suffer, but our future generations will also suffer. He lavishes His unfailing love on those who love Him and obey His commands for thousands of generations, but He does not hesitate to punish and destroy those who reject Him (Deuteronomy 7: 9-11).

Yahweh loves those who love and obey Him and only Him! (Deut 5:10). If you obey, you will *enjoy* a long life (Deuteronomy 6:2). That word 'enjoy' is so powerful and makes all the difference. What good is a long life if there is no joy?

Yahweh is the one true Creator in both Heaven and Earth, and there is no other! If you obey all His decrees and commands, all will be well with you and your children. You will enjoy a long life (Deuteronomy 4:39-40).

> *But seek first His Kingdom and His righteousness, and all these things will be given to you as well.* —Matthew 6:33

> *In order to obey the instructions of Yahweh your Creator which I am giving you, do not add to what I am saying, and do not subtract from it.* —Deuteronomy 4:2

After traveling all over the world, I've seen various eating customs and traditions, and the majority of them are breaking the command to keep our temples (our bodies) clean and pure. People are destroying their temples with every abomination to their lives. The most often used weapon to destroy the vessels Yahweh has given them is eating!

> *Hear, oh earth! I am going to bring disaster on this people; it is the consequence of their own way of thinking; for they pay no attention to My words; and as for My Torah, they reject it.* —Jeremiah 6:19

I created this book to reveal to everybody what the Scriptures have said about our health and also how we should eat: not only the type of food that is good for us, but when, why, and how to consume it, as well as what foods to avoid.

No matter what your situation, you can change your ways and begin to eat more along the lines Scripture guides us toward. No matter how far you may have backslidden from the instruction guide, it is not too late to start doing what is right. I've seen people with the worst diseases overcome their health issues by using the principles herein.

I have started a ministry based on these principles, Torah Life Ministries. With this ministry, it is my passion to reveal to believers all around the world that they must take care of their health, and they need to eat more healthfully. Another branch of this ministry is to teach the nonbelievers of this world who already know about eating healthfully that we have a Maker of all things. The food they are eating and the world we live in all come from

Yahweh, and no matter how much good food we consume, we must confess Yeshua is Messiah if we want to be saved.

People ask me which part of my ministry is the more challenging. A simple answer is, "It is easier to change a man's religion than to change a man's diet." Whoever you may be reading this book, I am not trying to change your ways or convert you to something you are not ready for. I only want you to understand that wherever you are, there is a more excellent way.

Notes to the Reader

How to Read This Book

The material in this book is separated into different parts to simplify its message. Although you may be tempted to skip right to the recipes or read the chapters haphazardly, the book was written to be read in order. I prayerfully designed the book so you can receive the most benefit from it in the order in which it is presented. It is important to understand each concept without missing anything before moving along to the next one.

Biblical Names

In this book, I use the true names of our Creator and His Son. Yahweh (YHWH) is the name of our Heavenly Father, and His Son's name is Yeshua. Yeshua means 'Yahweh's salvation'.

To help you understand and follow the pattern of names I use, I have alerted you by writing 'Yahweh (The Creator, commonly called God, Lord, Adonai)' and 'Yeshua (Our Messiah commonly called Jesus)' when these names first occur in the introduction. The rest of the book will not have '(God, Lord, Adonai)' or '(Jesus)' following the true name. The true names will also be substituted in biblical quotations wherever God, Lord, Adonai and Jesus are used in the cited translation's text. If you are interested in more information about the true names, you may also search the internet or contact me via my website www.torahlifeministries.com.

For better understanding, I also translated the following in certain texts: 'Lord your God' has been translated to 'Yahweh your Creator'. The Hebrew word *Mitzvot* has been translated to 'instructions'. Holy Spirit has been changed to Set-apart Spirit, or *Ruach haQodesh* in Hebrew.

Unless otherwise noted, all scriptural translations are from the Complete Jewish Bible, translated by David H. Stern. Other translations quoted and referenced herein are the New International Version (NIV), New Living Translation (NLT), the King James Version (KJV), and the New King James Version (NKJV).

Law versus Grace

Many Christians say they are saved by grace, so they no longer need to follow the law. This whole issue of law vs. grace has arisen because of a mistranslation of scripture.

In the original writings, the word 'law' as we know it was not there. Instead it said 'Torah'. Many people think the word 'Torah' means 'law', but it doesn't. It means 'guidelines' or 'instructions'. The will of Yahweh should be the foundation of our faith. To keep his Torah on our heart and in our actions should mean everything to us.

Yeshua did not do away with the instructions and guidelines of Yahweh. He came to serve as an example for us about how to achieve His Father's will. By our own strength, we cannot achieve perfection; but by His spirit, we can do all things in Him who strengthens us. Anytime we have not achieved His will, the blood of Yeshua carries us in those times we fall down, as long as our hearts and intentions are in the right place.

However, we are not healed by His stripes if we do not seek His will. If you want to have the blessing of health, follow the role model Yeshua set. That is why He is known as the Living Torah.

The word 'Torah' refers to the first five books of the Scriptures: Genesis, Exodus, Leviticus, Numbers and Deuteronomy. These books are the foundation of the Scriptures.

I also want to make it clear that no matter how much we are obedient to Yahweh's Torah, salvation comes only by the blood of the Messiah Yeshua. However, we must always remember He gave us the Torah to remain safe, healthy, and be blessed. The more obedient we are to His Torah, the more blessings we will receive.

In the subsequent text and scriptures in this book, I have replaced the often misquoted word 'law' with 'Torah' as needed in order to clear up confusion.

PART 1

My Commandments Are Not Burdensome. The Wise Shall Prosper.

CHAPTER 1

From Disease to Wellness:
Your Words Are Healing to All My Flesh.

I will never forget Your commandments, for You have used them to restore my joy and health. —Psalm 119:93 [NLT]

How I Healed from an Incurable Disease

Growing up in Brooklyn, New York, I had everything available to me in excess. My teenage wisdom kept me from making the wrong choices when it came to things like drugs and gangs, but I had no idea what damage I was causing to my body with my diet.

Here are some reasons why I had no idea that I was eating a harmful diet:

- My parents fed me common foods that everyone else was consuming.
- The teachers in school never taught me about healthful eating.
- Stores near my house were selling the foods.
- No doctor ever told me I had to be careful of what I ate.
- No one ever told me what food was healthful or not healthful. In fact, no one ever told me that food can cause disease. So I never put any connection between food and health.

When I was young, my friends used to say I had a stomach of iron because I could eat anything and not get sick. Girls used to get upset at me because I could consume as much as I wanted and not put on weight. I thought I was just lucky, so this led me to eat whatever food I wanted to, as much as I wanted to, and whenever I wanted to.

The only time my dad would mention food to me was when

he would say, "I'm going to the supermarket; what would you like me to buy you?" And the only time my mom would mention food was, "What would you like me to make for dinner tonight?"

Now I realize that the only reason I didn't get very sick when I was younger was because when we are young, we can eat just about anything and feel okay; but as we get older, what we consumed when we were younger catches up to us.

Reflecting back, I can recall this was the average diet for me:

Wake up:
    Four frozen waffles, toasted, with a load of sugary "syrup"
    A few bowls of cereal
Morning snack:
    Donuts or cookies
Lunch:
    Pizza, hotdog, or hamburger with soda
Afternoon snack:
    Cookies, cakes, candy, and more soda
Dinner:
    Chinese food, pizza, potato chips, and more soda
After dinner snack:
    Cake or cookies and more soda
Before bed:
    Soda or fruit juice drink (not fresh juice)

Notice I didn't have any produce at all in my diet. Also notice that this is the diet common to most people today. But back then, I didn't have any reason to worry about getting sick because I felt great, looked great, and lived great.

Then as I got older, I wanted to be able to be a winner when competing in sports, so I got involved with working out in a gym and reading bodybuilding magazines. Amongst all my friends growing up, I was the one who did everything to take care of my body. While they were playing sports, I was exercising in a gym. While they were reading magazines about cars, girls, and money, I was reading bodybuilding magazines. I wanted to be fit and healthy, and I thought I was. I was able to run the fastest, lift the most, and last the longest when up against most of my friends in competition.

I was sure my diet in my teenage years was much better:

Wake up:
    Bagel with bacon and cheese
    Scrambled eggs
    Orange juice
Morning snack:
    Protein shake and muffin
Lunch:
    Pasta with meatballs, french fries with soda
Evening snack:
    Ice cream or cookies
Supper:
    Steak or some other meat with soda
Before sleeping:
    Fruit juice

So that was my healthy diet growing up. Look familiar?

I was feeling great, so I had nothing to worry about. It seemed as if I had more energy than ever and was able to do more than anyone else.

Other than my diet, here's how I was living when I was nineteen years old:

5:00 a.m. — Wake up and take a train to New York City to the gym before work.
6:00 a.m. — Get to the gym and work out.
7:00 a.m. — Get to work.
5:00 p.m. — Leave work and take a train to college.
6:30 p.m. — Get to college.
9:30 p.m. — Leave college.
10:30 p.m. — Get home from college.
11:00 p.m. — Eat and watch TV for two hours.
1:00 a.m. — Go to sleep.

But everything was fine. I felt great, and I had so much energy. I never did like coffee, so I knew it was not stimulation I was running on. Oh, did I mention that all that soda I was drinking was called "Jolt!"? Just in case you've never heard of that, that's soda with like five times the caffeine of regular soda.

At age twenty, my health hit a brick wall. I started moving more slowly, my 30-inch waste was now 33 inches (but I was able to hide it well with my clothes), and I started to get bad stomachaches. Finally, I was home watching television one night when I got some bad stomach pains. I rushed to the bathroom. After I was in there for a while, the bowl filled with blood.

I was scared but didn't tell anyone, so I could wait and see if it was a one-time thing. It kept getting worse. My weight went from 160 to 120 in a few days. I finally went to the doctor, and she told me it seems I had food poisoning. What, are you kidding me? I knew it was more than that! After more time with the doctor running a bunch of tests, I was diagnosed with inflammatory bowel disease (also known as Crohn's disease, or ulcerative colitis), a deadly affliction.

The doctor told me there was no cure for my illness. She told me I was at high risk for colon cancer — at 20 years old! — and I had to take drugs for the rest of my life.

I took the drugs and did everything the doctor told me, but I wasn't getting better. I was getting worse. So I figured she wasn't a good doctor. I went to other doctors and did everything they told me to do. Still I was getting worse. I experienced side effects from the many drugs I was taking that were worse than the illness I was trying to control. I finally realized that the doctors didn't have the answers I was able to deal with, so I had to look elsewhere.

I read somewhere that diet had a lot to do with my illness, and it can be cured. I thought this can't be my cure because I was already eating a great diet. When I saw the list of foods to avoid, I realized that was my diet! As I eliminated those foods from my diet, I felt better and better. I still was not completely healed. I replaced all the foods that I eliminated from my diet with what I thought were more healthful choices. This was my new healthier diet:

Wake up:
> Tofu pancakes with organic syrup
> Orange juice (not fresh squeezed)
> Soy or rice milk

Mid-morning snack:
> Organic cookies or soy muffin

Lunch:
> Frozen soy pizza or soy burgers
> Fruit-sweetened soda

Afternoon snack:
> Soy ice cream

Dinner:
> Pasta and wheat bread

Snack before going to sleep:
> Soy milk with organic cake

A big improvement, huh? Today I know many people who add the word 'organic' or 'soy' to the same foods they were eating before and think they are now living healthfully. I thought the same thing, until...

To reduce the stress in my life, I moved from New York to West Palm Beach, Florida, at 23. I ended up moving not too far from a place called Hippocrates Health Institute. It's a natural health spa where people cleanse and strengthen so the body can heal from all types of so-called incurable diseases that the medical doctors have no answer for. I immediately began their program, switching my diet to a vegan diet consisting of 100% raw, ripe, fresh, organic fruits, vegetables, nuts, and seeds — and stopped overeating.

I called my doctor in New York City to make sure it was okay. When she told me, "No, it is very bad for you to eat that way," I knew I was on the right track.

I was amazed at how quickly my health returned. I was completely healed in no time. This led me to simplify all areas of my life. With my new understanding of "less is more," I left my office job and wrote some books about my story and the Hippocrates program. Now I spend my life traveling, giving lectures about health, and living simply all over the world.

It wasn't until years later that I was led to read the Scriptures for the first time and nearly fell out of my chair. You see, years ago when I was sitting in a waiting room office, someone told me to read the Scriptures, and I could be healed. I said no, thanks; I don't need that book.

Well, once I started to read it many years later, I saw that the diet suggestions in the Scriptures that Yahweh told us is medicine for us, is very close to the Hippocrates diet. I could have saved so much time and spared myself from so much pain if I had discovered this message years earlier.

But Yahweh had His timing for a reason, and I am so thrilled about where He has brought me today. Because of what I went though, I have such a passion and desire to learn more about the Scriptures and help people heal from their illnesses.

My life is now dedicated to studying and living according to the Scriptures and to developing my relationship with Yahweh. It is my prayer to help as many people as possible see the amazing health message of the Scriptures and to help them get to know and understand their Creator.

I am so excited that even though we live in a time where more people than ever before are living against the instructions found in the Scriptures, many people are looking more to Yahweh for the answers they couldn't find anywhere else. Today, the excessive number of choices available to us has confused many about whom to turn to when they have no hope left. This has resulted in the world's current tragic condition, especially when it comes to health. But many find Yahweh because of their trials.

I believe the Scriptures provide simple answers to keep us safe and get us back to a healthy state. I wrote this book to help everyone see that we truly have a Creator, and He wants the best for us. We just have to listen and believe. Following His directions is the only way we can truly be healthy in this world! When deeply understood and applied to our lives, the Scriptures give us the guidelines we need to stay healthy and fit and live a long and fulfilled life. May this book help you realize that!

It is my prayer that all people be blessed to fall in love with

Yahweh, who has lovingly revealed through His Word what is best for our health and well-being.

The more I study and pray about the Scriptures, the more I see how Yahweh has given us instructions for how to stay healthy physically, emotionally, and spiritually. I also realize more clearly why people suffer with disease.

I have given hundreds of presentations on the healing message of the Scriptures, and people are getting the point! Others have overlooked and rejected this information before making any attempt to confirm it. Instead, they choose that which will cause disease. A majority of us reject this knowledge willingly; however, many have simply been deceived. Lack of knowledge and laziness are often reasons why people continue to stay addicted to an unhealthy lifestyle. The great news is that more information is available than ever before to help guide people back in the right direction. It's such an exciting time to see people restoring their relationships with our heavenly King, Yahweh.

I present this message because our heavenly Father Yahweh has blessed me with insight about this subject and because it worked in my life, restoring me to health! I want to share this understanding with all who seek His will. Once the blessings are received by applying the instructions, your health will improve, and your faith will grow. I can't think of anything else that can be more encouraging.

The information I present duplicates the instructions Yahweh has given us in His great guidebook, the Scriptures. Since the Scriptures are rarely read in their entirety, the writings in my book may seem to be different from what you have been trained to believe. However, if you simply read the Word, you will find that I have kept the context of the message of Yahweh. It would be wise to study the points covered. When you adjust your actions to go along with this guide, you will be blessed by Yahweh.

Many brothers and sisters who truly have a heart for Yeshua are just as sick as nonbelievers. Yahweh wants better for us, and we have His instructions to reverse this unfortunate trend that is taking place. We need to have all people who preach the Word of the Scriptures stick to what it says, without trying to replace this important information for any reason.

As believers, we need to study and research what we are being taught to make sure it goes along with what the Scriptures say. As long as we consistently study the Word, no one will be able to mislead or deceive us. Good-hearted people should be blessed with good-hearted teachers who teach the Word of Yahweh. If we do that, we can all be blessed with great health.

Read Scripture daily and take action to follow the instructions. If you do, you will stay healthy, and there will be very little need for healing prayers. Instead, we will have more praising prayers for our great health. Hallelu-Yah!

Our comfort zone should go along with Yahweh's Word one hundred percent. We have to avoid and eliminate any lack of faith, man-made traditions, and pagan customs that have crept into teachings of Scripture over the years. We need to get back to the pure essence of His beautiful Word without any dirt thrown in. Even if we have become accustomed to — or even addicted to — living more in accordance with the world than with the Scriptures, it's time to clean up and experience the true beauty and joy of Yahweh's pure teachings and customs. When you do, any pain you suffer will be reversed and turned into joy.

In this book, I am going to introduce you to Yahweh's healing medicine. It is written to all those who want to experience Yahweh's healing touch and blessing of good health. Put the comforts of this world aside, and find comfort in the true Word of Yahweh. Once you do that, you will experience health according to the Scriptures.

Hallelu-Yah!

CHAPTER 2

Keep Your Word:
Commit Yourself to His Instructions

As for Me — I am herewith establishing My covenant with you, with your descendants after you. —Genesis 9:9

The Scriptures, as we know them today, have many words, names, and meanings that are different from what was in the original text. For example, today we say Old Testament and New Testament. The true meanings of these words are Old Covenant and New Covenant. It all comes down to the word 'covenant'. The word 'covenant' means 'promise'.

A covenant is a promise, a pact between two people or groups of people. Today, a promise means very little without signed documentation to back it up. Someone's word alone will not stand in the court system of today. In the ancient times of the Scriptures, it was very different. A covenant, or promise, meant everything. Their word was their bond. If it was ever broken, people knew there would be consequences not only by the law of the land, but also spiritually. For this reason, before people gave their word, they put much thought to it if they were wise; and once they gave their word, they did everything possible to keep it.

Offer thanksgiving as your sacrifice to Yahweh, pay your vows to the Most High. —Psalms 50:14

The Scriptures present the historical story about a covenant or promise between Yahweh and mankind. That promise is everlasting and will always be binding. The agreement is, "as long as we put our best effort into pleasing Yahweh, Yahweh will be happy and take care of us." Only Yahweh can know if we are making our best effort to keep our end of the deal. We can deceive man, but we can never deceive Yahweh. With thorough study, one will see the same promise in both the Old and New Covenant. We are also given the answer of how to please Yahweh — by listening and obeying His Word.

> *When a man makes a vow to Yahweh or formally obligates himself by swearing an oath, he is not to break his word but is to do everything he said he would do.* —Numbers 30:2

From now on instead of focusing on two covenants, an old and a new, understand that there is only one major promise, not two. A clearer way to state it would be to call them the Old Covenant and the Reminded Covenant, because what is commonly referred to today as the New Covenant or New Testament is just a reminder of the original promise Yahweh made with our fathers that we seem to have forgotten.

Yeshua means 'salvation' and was mentioned many times in the original promise. There is nothing new about *Him*. The message would be much clearer if we never again printed the Scriptures with a page separating the Old and New Covenants. In both covenants, Yeshua has always been the only way to our salvation. The only difference is that in the Old Covenant, man looked forward (towards the future) to the sacrifice of Yeshua by faith, along with his offerings and obedience to His commands. By contrast, today — after His sacrifice — we look back at what Yeshua did for us in His death. Thus, we are still to walk in obedience with strong faith. As long as our hearts are faithful, our actions will be obedient in either case.

> *Just as water reflects the face, so one human heart reflects another.*
> —Proverbs 27:19

When Yahweh spoke to Abraham, Isaac, and Jacob, He made a covenant with them and kept His word. Yahweh will never break His side of the deal because Yahweh will never lie to us. On the other hand, man has broken his side of the deal many times and continues to do so. Yahweh sets an example for man that no matter what the circumstances, we should never break our word.

There is much talk today about the Commandment that says

we should not lie or give false testimony. I think the real meaning of the Commandment is that we should not break our word, or promise. Technically, they may both mean the same thing, but it has been shown over and over again that there can be no peace in the land or within our physical bodies if we cannot trust one another.

We shouldn't lie, but there are certain exceptions in the Scriptures where even the most righteous people would lie to save a life, and it seemed fine according to Yahweh. The fruit of those people support that. A lie to save a righteous person is not the same as giving your word and not following through.

Joshua, one of the most righteous people in the Scriptures, understood the value of a covenant. In Joshua 6:22, he told his two spies to keep their promise to bring Rahab and her family to a safe place near the camp of Israel, even though Rahab had lied to save them (in Joshua 2).

Later in the book of Joshua, we find another example of the righteousness of Joshua and the importance of keeping his word.

> *But when the inhabitants of Gibeon heard what Joshua had done to Jericho and Ai,*
> *they developed a clever deception.* —Joshua 9:3-4

After this deception by the people of Gibeon, Joshua foolishly made covenant with them to let them live and made a peace treaty with them that they wouldn't be killed (Joshua 9:15). Once the Jewish leaders found out that they had been deceived, they were very angry but still knew that they couldn't go back on their word:

> *However, the leaders replied to the whole community, "We have sworn to them by Yahweh, the Creator of Israel; so we can't touch them.*
> *Here is what we will do to them: we will let them live, so that Yahweh's anger will not be on us because of the oath we swore to them."* —Joshua 9:19-20

In the book of Samuel, Saul later broke this promise when he killed many Gibeonites. Because of this broken covenant, there was famine in the days of David for three years (2 Samuel 21:1). This is just one powerful example of the importance of a covenant, that it is forever, and there are consequences for breaking it.

> *A curse on anyone who does not pay attention to the words of this covenant.* —Jeremiah 11:3

Man began to suffer with disease and other consequences after Adam broke the covenant with Yahweh in the Garden of Eden (Genesis 3:6). Man has been cursed since (Genesis 3:16-17). At some point in every person's life, Adam's disobedience has tormented us.

Many scriptures show that we will suffer if we displease Yahweh. Even David, one of the most righteous servants, suffered because of his disobedience to Yahweh (adultery and murder). No one is released from this eternal covenant. Just like Adam and Eve and just like David, we suffer for our sin today.

Accepting Yeshua into our hearts doesn't excuse us from the covenant; it makes us more accountable. When we accept Yeshua into our hearts, we are personally renewing the covenant our fathers made with Yahweh to live according to His Word and do things that will please Him, to love the things He loves and to hate the things that He hates. We are admitting that we know and accept the terms and are accountable to live righteous lives.

Yahweh knew that because of our weakness of the flesh, people would blame their troubles and sins on their parents, taking no responsibility for their own actions. So that we will not have this excuse to fall back on, Yahweh has made a newer covenant (renewed promise) to make us responsible for our own actions (Jeremiah 31:31-34); but because of His kindness, He gave us a Helper to achieve the goal. He gave us His Son Yeshua, and Yeshua gave us the Set-apart Spirit (Holy Spirit). Hallelu-Yah!

It brings me such joy to know that I can personally renew the promise that our fathers have drifted away from and break this chain of disobedience. It brings me even more joy to know that Yahweh can look beyond our transgressions and take the most unrighteous man and make him righteous. Shaul (the apostle Paul) is a great example. If Yahweh can forgive such a misguided soul as Shaul and turn his life around to use him in such a powerful way, then no matter how far we have drifted from the covenant, there is always hope for us. No matter how much we have suffered for our iniquities and transgressions, relief is always possible. No matter how sick or diseased you might be, healing is still possible! Hallelu-Yah!

The overall message Yeshua preached was, "Return to the promise your fathers made with Yahweh, and you will no longer commit and suffer from iniquity, and your transgressions will be forgiven" (Matthew 4:17).

Our focus must always be in the right place (on Yeshua); otherwise, it is very easy for us to be led astray. Let Yahweh control your thinking, and you will be strong and persevere always, regardless of what you go through.

> *So when you make a promise to Yahweh, don't delay in following through, for Yahweh takes no pleasure in fools. Keep all the promises you make to Him.*
>
> *It is better to say nothing than to promise something that you don't follow through on.* —Ecclesiastes 5:4-5 [NLT]

A History Lesson

Because most people today have not even read the Scriptures, including most believers, I feel it is important to give a brief history lesson. The Torah is often referred to as law, but it really means guidelines, or teachings (see Notes to the Reader). As revealed in the Scriptures, it is a good, right, and perfect system of moral principles that reflects Yahweh's character and serves as a means of expressing His love toward man. The principles of the Scriptures teach man how to properly worship Yahweh, how to love his fellow man, how to live life abundantly, and at the same time, how to prepare for an eternal spiritual life. These principles and guidelines are represented in both the Old and New Covenants and are expressed by both physical actions and spiritual motivations.

Many people overlook the fact that the original Ten Commandments were written by the hand of Yahweh, and that the Scriptures are a compilation of books filled with stories and examples of what happened to people when they kept or broke Yahweh's personal, handwritten words. Because many people were sinning in their hearts, Yahweh's new approach was to write the covenant on our hearts and in our minds (Hebrews 8:7-11). Of course this is not literal; no one thinks that if we cut open our chest, we would see the Ten Commandments written on our beating hearts. Yahweh desires that the "Ten Commandments" be such an integral part of our being (i.e., be written on our hearts and in our minds) that we would truly keep them.

Many people today will accept Yeshua as the Messiah with their lips but still choose not to change their ways of living, committing the same wickedness against Yahweh that their fathers committed and continuing to go back on their promise. They have been given a clause in the original contract to be released from their fathers' sins, but then they commit their own sins. This is a common reason sickness and disease continue to stay in their lives, and many generations of a family suffer from common illnesses. There is so much sickness in assemblies today, and a big reason is because people are living lives with pagan practices on a daily basis — either wittingly or unwittingly.

After the Commandments were written by Yahweh, all the texts in the Scriptures were written by man inspired by the Set-apart Spirit (2 Peter 1:21). It all points to showing us how to please Yahweh by following the agreement that came from His own hand! We must consistently give our best effort to please Him. That is the real covenant our fathers made with *Him*.

CHAPTER 3

Freedom:
The Truth Shall Set You Free

But if you refuse to pay attention to what Yahweh your Creator says, and do not observe and obey all His Torah and regulations which I am giving you today, then all the following curses will be yours in abundance. —Deuteronomy 28:15

Yahweh will strike you down with wasting diseases, fever, inflammation, fiery heat, drought, blasting winds and mildew; and they will pursue you until you perish. —Deuteronomy 28:22

Once you accept Yeshua, it is the beginning of a beautiful new life. Action will follow your heart's desire to have Yahweh's salvation. The Scriptures are filled with guidelines that we should willingly desire to uphold. Read Psalms 119 and see the importance of following Yahweh's instructions. How you live will be observed by many. Your new actions will become your greatest witness.

The best way to confirm what Yahweh desires is to study His guide. The Scriptures tell us all about Him and what He wants for us. It also tells us how to achieve a disease-free, joyful life.

Now that you have decided to join Yahweh's kingdom, your passion to learn more about Yahweh should always be at high levels. We are now part of Yahweh's kingdom and set apart for a purpose. We will be different from the worldly people who could care less about Yahweh.

The Scriptures contain the most vital information for survival, and most people have chosen never to read the whole book. It is common that the only time people open the Scriptures is once a week in church or when they want to quickly look up a single verse.

Amongst all the distractions in today's world, we should set time apart daily to get to know about Him! Feeding your body with daily spiritual food is the best nourishment you can give your body. If you do not have time to study the Word of Yahweh at home, read it in public! There is no reason to hide your passion to acquire this vital information.

Take every opportunity you have to read it. Waiting in line at the store (instead of reading the trashy gossip magazines near the counter), waiting for the bus, or waiting in waiting rooms, and so on, you have many opportunities to find time to read the Scriptures. Let people know how much it means to you. When you give someone a greeting, wave the Scriptures at him or her. Take it to work and everywhere you go. People will get the picture without your saying a word.

In this backwards world today, we may easily be called crazy if our actions follow the instructions of Yahweh: dressing, speaking, and eating in a righteous way according to the way Yahweh commands us. Well, our great Doctor in heaven will find joy in your not conforming to this world, and He will bless you with joy and the pain-free life that you desire.

We have to be willing to give up every earthly material thing to receive this blessing from Yahweh, not holding things so dear to our heart that they become idols in our lives. The good news is that it is possible to live in paradise in the midst of our shameful culture. This doesn't mean Yahweh will take everything away from you and leave you empty; it means you will be full if you stick to the covenant!

We need to wake up and stop hoping for healing. We need to read, believe, obey, and experience the healing. After that, we need to be doctors and give this healing knowledge to others who are sick. Believers and nonbelievers alike need the medicine of the Word. The Scriptures are strictly for the benefit of man, and anyone who uses them wisely will assure himself of the best health possible from an emotional, mental, and physical standpoint.

Yeshua commands that we take the good news to every person on this earth. Many people of the past, including Yeshua, were despised, rejected, hated, mocked, ridiculed, and reproached for teaching the Word. I myself have seen firsthand how people react when I take out my Scriptures or even mention the Word. To me it brings joy! I know the enemy hates the Word of Yahweh. The Word is my protection, my medicine.

Many times in Scripture the word 'evil' can be replaced with the word 'disease'. Often they have the same meaning in different scriptures. If we want to heal our diseases, we have to get the evil out. The Scriptures is a book of opposites. We have blessings versus curses, good versus evil, life versus death, and health versus disease. You cannot have both in your life at the same time. You have one or the other. If you keep your end of the promise, you will have good, blessings, health, and life. Continue to break the covenant, and you will have evil, curses, sickness, disease, and death.

Many righteous people have missed important messages in Scripture, many of them about health, but more importantly about the promise and the responsibility of keeping our end of the deal. On Yahweh's side of the deal, He promises us a healthy, long life without sickness or disease. On our side of the deal, we please Him. We should be very extreme to make sure we are pleasing Him. Hallelu-Yah!

You will know the truth, and the truth shall set you free. —John 8:32

Yahweh has blessed us with the freedom to choose our paths and make our own choices. Once you truly know Yahweh, deciding to follow the covenant will not be a difficult choice. You will excitedly enjoy learning and obeying His Word. To accept His covenant and to learn and meditate on His Word day and night are the most exciting things you can ever do in your life. Having true faith in and obeying Yahweh's guide will free us from the entrapment of all evil (sin, sickness, and disease).

During the ministry of Yeshua, He said several times, "Drop everything and follow me right now." It is the most freeing feeling to know you can do that and not have to worry about anything because Yahweh will take care of you as long as you stick to your end of the promise and live by His guide.

In 1 Peter 2:16, we are told that we are free as people, yet that we should not use this freedom as an excuse to do evil, but rather to become joyful slaves to Yahweh. If we are a true believer and have tremendous faith, we joyfully become a servant to Yahweh's Word. Yahweh will be our commander because we choose Him and His path for us. We make the decision to listen and obey His Word because we have faith. This is the best place we can be. Nothing will satisfy us more.

Being a slave to Yahweh's Word does not trap us. It frees us. Use your freedom as a tool for a life of exuberant service. It's the foundation that Yahweh gives to us to reach our highest potential. Our newfound freedom should help us reach for the best Yahweh has for us. Just make sure that what you seek is of Yahweh's will.

When the apostle Paul prayed or said things about what he wanted, he always prefaced it with "if it be Yahweh's will." That is what we should do also each time we pray. We have to believe and trust that Yahweh wants what's best for us always, because He does! That's so exciting to know, I get chills just thinking about it. Hallelu-Yah!

Any struggles I have to go through for Yahweh are well worth it. Even though Yahweh will forgive us if our heart is for Him, we must never take that for granted and always strive to be perfect. With one slip-up, we can reap the results.

Take for example how righteous Joshua was: He was chosen by Yahweh (through Moses) and obeyed and kept his promises. However, as righteous as Joshua was, we can see how even the most righteous among us can make errors in judgment against Yahweh. Joshua didn't lie or break his promises, but in Joshua 9:14, Joshua and the Israelites made a big error in answering and giving their word before consulting Yahweh: "So the Israelites examined their food, but they did not consult Yahweh."

We need to be very careful when we pray. Yahweh knows what has to be done and when it has to be done. He just wants us to listen, obey, and be thankful. A good way to pray would be as Yahweh told us to pray, for wisdom, knowledge, and strength.

Wisdom: What needs to be done? What is your will for me?

Knowledge: What is the best way to do it? How to get it done? Strength: Give me strength to do the things you ask me to do.

I never want to change Yahweh's will for my path in life, so I only ask Him for things if it be His will. You can miss accomplishing His will if you go against His answers to your prayers.

We need to be very careful what we pray for. Yahweh has a perfect will for each of us, but if we keep praying and asking Him for something different, He may very well answer our prayers even though it goes against His will for our lives.

I always respect a company or business that will pray before each business day about each important decision regarding the direction the company should take on issues. But I respect more those companies that hear and obey the reply. I can tell which companies do this, based on the fact that Yahweh would never ask us to do something that wasn't in His Scriptures. Just as a company will be blessed or cursed by its daily practices, so too will our lives be blessed or cursed according to our own daily practices.

It is Yahweh's will for us to follow the guide He has laid out for us in the Scriptures. When it comes to diet, Yahweh has given us instructions regarding what foods to eat. He has freely given us food that tastes delicious. But man spends time and money finding ways to process the food so that by the time we get it, it is as far as possible from the original form in which Yahweh wanted for us to eat it.

It is so common to live against the guide of Yahweh in today's world that sometimes it seems people do things just to go opposite of Yahweh's will. It is Yahweh's will for us not to be sick, not to experience disease, and to live long, healthy lives. Instead, people today choose sickness, disease, and shortened lives. That's what we ask for when we say we want to do it our own way without Yahweh. As believers, we don't have to worry about this situation so long as His commands are written on our hearts. Hallelu-Yah!

Up to now in this book about health, I've mentioned many nondietary things that affect our health and also discussed why so many believers are sick. When you picked up this book, many of you might have thought I was going to speak only about diet, because most books about health focus only on food. There is a big connection between the quality of the food you consume and your health; however, this book also covers important non-food-related aspects of health. I want everyone to learn why people suffer from disease and how to overcome it. My goal is to increase your awareness of some very important facts about why we suffer.

Health is more than just diet alone. We need to realize that:

1. If we have broken our promise, we must get back to the guide of Yahweh if we want our health to return. No matter how long you have been a believer, you need to revisit the covenant and make sure you are keeping your side of the deal.

2. If we keep our promise, we will be blessed with great health and joy in our lives.

3. We have to trust and have faith in Yahweh in order to receive His blessings!

These concepts are the foundation of a healthy life, and it's time we get a solid foundation!

Read the Scriptures many times, over and over again. Each time something new will jump out at you. As you make these new discoveries, pleasing Yahweh will become easier and easier. Make reading the Word of Yahweh an important daily task. Take time to study and pray about what you read, becoming more familiar with Yahweh and the promise.

Habit versus Addiction

Habit: Doing something that you enjoy on a regular basis, but when you find out it is unhealthful or bad, you stop it. You break that habit.

Addiction: Doing something you enjoy on a regular basis, but when you find out it is unhealthful or bad, you make excuses to keep doing it.

We must change our addictions to habits and break them. People today are addicted to pleasing their flesh and not hearing the Word of Yahweh. They are addicted to eating a diet against what the Scriptures tell us is wise and good for us and living lives against the principles of the Scriptures. Most people today are seriously addicted to watching television — many hours each day — where ninety percent of the messages go against Yahweh's guide. This leads them to commit great abominations against Yahweh on a daily basis. Many of us become addicted to destructive things because we are too weak in the flesh alone (without the Set-apart Spirit and/or knowledge of Yahweh) to avoid them.

If most people took the time they spend watching television and instead read the Scriptures, they would be much stronger to resist temptation.

There are many other addictions that people have today, but because those addictions are so common in today's world, people just accept them as normal. It's time we stopped making excuses and get right with Yahweh. Instead of making excuses, people need to change their addictions to habits and break those habits. Then you can be on a path Yahweh chooses for you and start to receive and enjoy His blessings.

Hallelu-Yah!

CHAPTER 4

The Power of Adaptation:
Let Yahweh Transform You into a New Person.

In other words, do not let yourselves be conformed to the standards of the world. Instead, keep letting yourselves be transformed by the renewing of your minds; so that you will know what Yahweh wants and will agree that what He wants is good, satisfying and able to succeed. —Romans 12:2

We are wonderfully and amazingly built (Psalms 139:14). Because of this, we have the ability to adapt to various environments. This can be good or bad, depending on the environment. The friends and people we have fellowship with and spend our personal time with can have a big impact on our spiritual lives.

Emotionally, we can adapt to deal with the most unnatural, stressful situations; physically, we can adapt to eating a very unhealthful diet; and spiritually, we can adapt to living in a culture that is in spiritual darkness. Just because we have this ability to adapt doesn't mean that's what Yahweh wants for us. If we are adapting to an unhealthful environment, we may not feel the effects right away, but we will eventually become a victim to the negative things in our environment.

For example, take the air we're breathing. Most of us today are breathing poor-quality air without noticeable discomfort. If a healthy person were to be placed in the same poor air, it would seem intolerable to him. This adaptation is termed "immunity." According to this theory, man becomes immune to a condition or poison if it doesn't kill him on the spot. Such adaptation can occur only at the expense of the general depression of all vital functions. The adaptation necessarily becomes injurious if long continued or often repeated.

It is in this condition that people slowly get sicker and sicker while being treated for some "mysterious disease." There is no mystery at all. If you keep doing the same thing, you will keep getting the same result. Change your action until it agrees with Yahweh's Torah (the first five books of the Scriptures)!

The body is so perfectly equipped with the power of adaptation that it will adjust itself, in time, to tolerate an atmosphere so poisonous that it would sicken a vital, healthy man in a short time if he were suddenly exposed to it.

Due to the body's power of adaptation, people can live in constantly polluted air and suffer nothing more on the surface than coughs, colds, hay fever, sore throats, and other relatively mild ailments of the respiratory organs. Yet, they are dying inch by inch from the effects of that air and don't know it. Every sneeze, every cough, every cold, and every headache are the first warnings that you are diseased.

Just as the body has an amazing power to adapt to its outer environment, it also has the same capability for adapting emotionally and spiritually. Each day, people are getting more and more away from living lives at emotional peace, known in Hebrew as *shalom*. People seem comfortable in their comfort zones, but what people call "comfortable" today is far beyond what would have been considered stressful just a few years ago. People are getting so accustomed to the stress that they think it is gone, but it is not gone. They are learning how to accept it and live with it, but it is still creating disease inside. Man was never intended to live under the stressful situations that he is put under today on a daily basis.

It's a wonder to me how people can even survive without knowing Yahweh personally. But then again, it is no wonder that people are just barely surviving instead of thriving as we were meant to be. It is just a matter of time before people who have adapted to the stress have nervous breakdowns.

People are living so far away from the principles of the Torah and have gone so far in the opposite direction to worship idols in their lives that they have completely disrespected the one and only Creator Yahweh, by living directly against the way that is pleasing to Him. His warnings are being laughed at; His signs are being ignored. His history has been rejected and forgotten.

When people ask me why they are sick or have a disease, if I don't have a copy of this book to give them, I point them to Hosea 4:1-3. That scripture clearly gives us the answer:

> *Hear the Word of Yahweh, O People of Israel! Yahweh has filed a lawsuit against you, saying: There is no faithfulness, no kindness, and no knowledge of Yahweh in your land.*
>
> *You curse and lie and kill and steal and commit adultery. There is violence everywhere, with one murder after another.*
>
> *That is why your land is not producing. It is filled with sadness, and all living things are becoming sick and dying. Even the animals, birds, and fish have begun to disappear.* —Hosea 4:1-3 [NLT]

People have gotten used to living in the spiritual darkness and have thrown away the Light. In the stories of the Scriptures, we have seen what happened in the past when people adapted to a culture that rejects Yahweh. If we don't reject that culture's ways, we will continue to be sucked into it without even realizing it.

It would seem that Yahweh's mercy should bring people back to obeying his statutes and commands, choosing to turn their hearts toward Him. But the opposite has happened. Because of deception, pride, greed, and addictions, people are being pushed even further away. Masking their suffering with adaptation, justifying their disrespect with addiction, and blaming their disobedience on the enemy, people have taken advantage of Yahweh's kindness and are asking for trouble!

Most people don't understand what health is and what the body needs. They take poisonous remedies, further depressing their vital functions and suppressing their symptoms while they continue to ignore and/or defy Yahweh's instructions. They read self-help books for emotional comfort while acquiring eating disorders in the meantime and rejecting the best self-help book of all, the Scriptures. Spiritually they are misinformed and misled to follow other elohim (gods), leaving them lost and broken.

> *You were at ease in your wickedness, you thought, "No one sees me." Your "wisdom" and "knowledge" perverted you, as you thought to yourself, "I am important, and no one else."*

> *Yet disaster will befall you, and you won't know how to charm it away; calamity will come upon you, and you won't be able to turn it aside; ruin will overcome you, suddenly, before you know it.*
>
> *So for now, keep on with your powerful spells and your many occult practices; from childhood you have been working at them; maybe they will do you some good, maybe you will inspire terror!*
>
> *You are worn out with all your consultations — so let the astrologers and stargazers, the monthly horoscope-makers, come forward now and save you from the things that will come upon you!*
> —Isaiah 47:10-13

We want our bodies to react, not adapt, when we eat something unhealthful so they can warn us quickly, and we can avoid the problem foods in the future. If we avoid the mind-altering society and stay focused on the true way to live, the true path to follow, and the promise we have made with Yahweh, our minds will be sharp with wisdom instead of being filled with pride, and we will not be misled. If we talk to Yahweh on a consistent basis and stay focused on His Word and our promise, along with having faith in Him always, we will overcome all evil, sickness, and disease! We should no longer continue to adapt to the world and instead put all of our focus into adapting to the Word!

> *In that day He will be your sure foundation, providing a rich store of salvation, wisdom, and knowledge. The fear of Yahweh is the key to this treasure.* —Isaiah 33:6 [NLT]

> *The fear of Yahweh leads to life; one who has it is satisfied and rests untouched by evil.* —Proverbs 19:23

While we are on the subject of the power of adaptation, we cannot overlook the fact that people today are not led to read His Word, instead saying they are good people, so they will be fine.

"As long as I am a good person and do good things, Yahweh will give me good and bless me." That is what I hear most often from people who don't know Yahweh's Word or believe in His promise.

Many other popular religions around the world teach that.

That is not the message Yahweh teaches. The statement is true to a degree, as we will be blessed for following Yahweh's instructions, but following Yahweh's guide without accepting Yeshua as our Messiah is not going to do it. We must do more than just "good." The answer is to do good *and* accept Yeshua as your Messiah.

That brings up another question: what does *good* mean? Good to one person might not mean the same thing to another, and this is where much of the problem starts. People want to make up their own minds and live by their own feelings.

> *For the old nature wants what is contrary to the Spirit, and the Spirit wants what is contrary to the old nature. These oppose each other, so that you find yourselves unable to carry out your good intentions.* —Galatians 5:17

The same thing holds true about health. Health to one person can mean something completely different to another.

We can say the same thing about what the word 'moral' means. To come up with an answer to these questions, we all have to decide what our standard will be and stick to that decision always, no matter what happens in our lives. When we truly accept Yeshua as our Messiah and receive the Set-apart Spirit, it will not be burdensome to live our lives according to Yahweh's guide. Having faith in Yahweh will achieve our goals.

Living by what people in the world say is good, moral, and right, instead of what Yahweh's Word says, is a mistake. Yahweh's guide will always produce health, peace, and joy. The word of the world is determined by what is trendy or popular at that particular time and can never assure us of the outcome, but history shows it will usually end up in a result opposite to our goal. What is right is not always popular, and what is popular is not always right.

From a health standpoint, many people listen to what the world (media) says is healthy and then follow that advice. This is one reason the nations around the world who are not using the Word of Yahweh as their guide are much sicker than the ones that do.

> We need to understand, listen to, and obey Yahweh's Word always!
> *But these people mock and curse the things they do not understand. Like animals, they do whatever their instincts tell them, and they bring about their own destruction.*
>
> *How terrible it will be for them! For they follow the evil example of Cain, who killed his brother. Like Balaam, they will do anything for money. And like Korah, they will perish because of their rebellion.*
> —Jude 1:10-11 [NLT]

Today there are people who attempt to live by the so-called law of attraction, believing that the way they act will determine what they get, regardless of what Yahweh or the world says. This might be the most popular way of thinking today in modern culture, but it is a very selfish way to live and cannot give us the health, peace, and joy Yahweh's Word can give us.

Instead of living according to the law of attraction, we should be living according to the Torah of Yahweh! There are people who will attack the rules of Yahweh, saying we are legalists if we strive to follow Yahweh's rules, but those same people have no issue with following the so-called law of attraction. Living by any law is being law-abiding, not "legalistic."

There is nothing wrong with living a lawful life according to the Scriptures as long as we understand we get into heaven not by our works, but only by accepting Yeshua. But if we accept Yeshua truly with our hearts, we will be happily following the Torah of Yahweh, because that is what Yeshua commanded us to do. Many of the prophets also tell us this is the way to live:

> *Those who love Your Torah have great peace; nothing makes them stumble.* —Psalms 119:165

> *But if a person looks closely into the perfect Torah, which gives freedom, and continues, becoming not a forgetful hearer but a doer of the work it requires, then he will be blessed in what he does.*
> —James 1:25

The wise way to decide what is good and right according to Yahweh's Word is to consult the great instruction guide, the Torah. The Torah tells us what is good and what is evil. It doesn't change according to the trends of this world. It is always the same no matter how we feel, and it always forgives us for our mistakes, working to our advantage. If we really want to define the word 'good', we must avoid the common scales that deceive and mislead us and use as our standard Yahweh's Word, the Scriptures.

This is why the Scriptures comprise the best health book ever written: it tells us what is truly healthful and unhealthful, or good and bad, when it comes to health. It also tells us how to deal with avoiding and healing sickness. On a much larger scale, it defines moral and immoral, curses and blessings, and ultimately life and death.

When It Comes to Health, What Are We Looking to Achieve?

When I asked the question and gave people a chance to really think about it, I found that all who put serious thought into it said the top three things they really were looking for are

- Pain-free lives (no painful disease)
- Shalom (emotional peace)
- Everlasting joy (continuous joy)

People don't mind disease, but they mind the pain that comes with it.

Many people today are attached to their diseases, and some even get benefits from the government, along with special attention from friends and family, but it's the pain and suffering that goes along with disease that people really want to recover from or avoid.

The word 'peace' in English is not necessarily the same word as 'shalom' (peace) in Hebrew. *Shalom* has much more meaning. It is an overall peace in the body. Emotional peace is also something we all want. It's a continuous state of emotional wellness. Having a close personal relationship with Yahweh will give shalom to someone. Just like any relationship, we must consistently work at it and nurture it always.

Happiness comes from the outside. When we are affected by something, or something happens, we become either happy or unhappy. However, joy comes from the inside and is constant. If you know Yahweh on a personal level and you know that you are seeking to please Him with all your heart, you will have everlasting joy. As long as we trust His Word and His promise, nothing can take away that joy. And as long as that relationship is strong, wanting to please Yahweh will be a joy, not a task.

Chapter 5

The Power of Temperance: Yahweh is Near to All Those Who Call Him.

Stay awake, and pray that you will not be put to the test — the spirit indeed is eager, but human nature is weak. —Matthew 26:41

Temperance — The Practice of Moderation

This chapter is about temperance. Temperance is the practice of moderation. I don't like to use the word 'moderation' because from my experience, people often use it to denote what they feel is moderate. Moderate to one person can be extreme to another. I think a better definition for temperance would be restraint or self-control, maybe even the opposite of excess. It might perhaps be moderation compared to what they were doing, but just lessening doesn't mean they are practicing temperance.

I find most people are addicted to excess in many areas of life. Temperance not only seems boring, but unattainable. I understand this thinking because I have met many sick people in my life, but I haven't met too many people my size and weight that ate more than I used to eat. I don't meet many people bigger than I who used to eat as much as I used to. I would say my life was a life of excess. It always had to be more. Temperance was the furthest thing from my mind.

Regarding nutrition, I couldn't understand how less could be better than more. So I would eat and eat and eat, not knowing the damage I was creating. All the extra stuff I was eating was going to waste, taking my body down with it.

I do understand and respect the fact that when it comes to chemistry and nutrition, there is no one amount for everyone. We each come in different sizes and weights. What is considered little for one person can be a lot for another. However, based on body type, age, current nutritional profile, climate, and physical condition, taking into account the quality of the food, there is a standard moderate amount for each of us.

This amount shouldn't be based on how we feel or what we believe, but purely on the fact that our bodies need a certain amount of nutrients to survive. Any amount above that is going to lessen the condition of our health. Many of us would be surprised to find out we are nowhere close to eating the amount we should, eating way in excess. Many are not surprised but simply don't care.

We also have to be careful not to decide how much we need based on our weight. Muscle weighs more than fat, so forget about that excuse or loophole. I had to mention that because when it comes to diet, it is a weird new teaching to claim this stored fat is good for us. It's not good if you are carrying around extra fat. It means you are taking in more than you need. The sign couldn't get more obvious than that. It becomes, is, and will always be, waste.

In his book *The Natural Food for Man*, Dr. Hereward Carrington said the following:

> Every individual should restrict himself to the smallest quantity that he finds, from careful investigation and experiment, will meet the wants of his system, knowing that whatever is more than this is harmful.

Luigi Cornaro was a man who lived 102 years. His secret for a long life was very simple:

> Man should live up to the simplicity dictated by nature, which teaches us to be content with little, and accustom ourselves to eat no more than is absolutely necessary to support life, remembering that all excess causes disease and leads to death.

The amazing thing about Mr. Cornaro is that when he was 35, he ate just as much as the average person of that time until he got very sick. The doctors told him he was not going to live long. So he started practicing temperance with his food and died at 102, in 1566!

Mr. Cornaro came to the same conclusion many other centenarians came to: If temperance has efficacy enough to heal the sick, it must also have the power to preserve us in health and strength.

All the major popular spiritual leaders in history teach temperance, especially when it comes to diet. Yeshua warned His disciples that a state of things would exist just prior to His second coming that would be very similar to that which preceded the flood. Eating and drinking would be carried to excess, and the world would be given up to greed.

My first two books spoke about the types of foods that are best for our bodies. They are raw, ripe, fresh, organic, living foods! However, when and how often we eat has just as much of an impact on our health, maybe even more. I know many people who eat lousy diets but don't overeat, and they seem to be doing somewhat okay. I also know a lot of people who eat more healthful foods but overeat, and they are not doing any better, in fact much worse in many cases.

Health doesn't begin with what we add to our diet, but with what we leave out. If overeating is causing us so many issues, doesn't it seem sensible and wise to stop overeating?

These are the two great evils to all men who live a free life; the one is troublesome and painful; the other, dreadful and insupportable, especially when they reflect on the errors to which this mortal life is subject, and on the vengeance which the justice of Yahweh is wont to take on sinners. Whereas, I, in my old age — praise to the Almighty — am exempt from these torments: from the first, because I cannot fall sick, having removed all the cause of illness by my regularity and moderation; from the other, that of death, because from so many years' experience, I have learned to obey reason; whereas, I not only think it a great folly to fear that which cannot be avoided, but likewise firmly expect some consolation,

from the grace of Messiah Yeshua, when I arrive at that period.
—Luigi Cornaro, from his book *Discourses on the Sober Life: How to Live to 100 Years.*

CHAPTER 6

The Scriptures:
Use Them or Lose Them!
The Teaching of His Word Gives Light!

Your word is a lamp to guide my feet and a light for my path.
—Psalms 119:105 [NLT]

Yeshua used the Torah as his guideline and standard. He lived according to the Torah and taught that the Torah should be man's guide and standard (Matthew 5:17, 12:50, 19:17). Without the Torah, one simply cannot tell the difference between what is good and what is evil. One would be left lost, just like people who choose to use the world's ways, the law of attraction, or their emotions as their guide. Without the Torah, you are walking in the dark with no light. The Torah is a light on a dark path.

The ancient Hebrews were the first to receive the written Torah from Moses. With Torah as their guide, they understood the important practices that must be observed to avoid disease and to stay healthy. They were given strict rules, or guidelines, and they took them very seriously. Some rebelled and suffered, but many followed the instructions in the Torah and were rewarded with great health and energy.

The daily health practices followed by the obedient Hebrews included

- Good hygiene
- Isolation of communicable diseases and their carriers
- Disinfection of all possibly contaminated articles
- Weekly rest and relaxation
- Hard work and exercise
- Good education and mental exercises to stay alert
- Rules regarding healthful food

Because of their obedience to the Word of Yahweh, the children of Israel were the healthiest people in ancient times. Keeping clean, bathing often, especially after touching something that might be dirty or carry germs, was of immense importance. People with contagious diseases were quarantined, and so were the people who touched them. As for treating sickness, the answers were sought once again in Yahweh's wisdom rather than in hospitals.

As for nutrition, Yahweh knew from the beginning exactly what the best diet would be for man, as stated in His Torah. By means of the Scriptures, Yahweh's health guidelines were passed down to the Hebrew people generation after generation. Thousands of years later, science is finally just starting to agree with many of those health guidelines found in the Scriptures. The dietary rules, strictly observed by the Jewish people during Old Testament times, allowed them to avoid and survive many plagues that afflicted people who didn't know about the Scriptures as an amazing health guide. The closer we adhere to His guidebook, the better health we'll have for it.

As long as people reject Yahweh's guide, they will suffer. Living according to man and not according to our Creator Yahweh will cause sickness in three dimensions:

1. Spiritually

When we live our lives according to the Torah, we see the positive outcomes, which build our faith and our strength. However, living according to the world's views and against Yahweh's views can weaken our faith and put us in danger when under spiritual attack. If we lose faith in Yahweh, it opens a door for the enemy to attack us spiritually.

2. Mentally

Living according to man and not according to Yahweh affects our thoughts, and doubt sets in. It is our thoughts that cause us to live against Yahweh, not the enemy, but we open the door for the enemy to make things worse if we lose focus.

3. Physically
Living according to man and not according to Yahweh brings disease and death to our bodies. It also seeks to convince us to act out our temptations. The enemy rejoices at seeing Yahweh's creations destroy themselves and then blame the results on the enemy. Do not give the enemy any reason to be joyful.

We can overcome or avoid these issues in the same three dimensions:

1. Spiritually
Have faith in Yahweh always and forever, no matter what happens. Read Psalms 1 every day and live according to what it says.

2. Mentally
Compare your thoughts to the Scriptures. Our thoughts should go along with Yahweh's guide.

3. Physically
Our actions will follow our hearts and will keep us from the dangers of this world that can harm us.

Yahweh's words must become so ingrained in our thinking, our hearts, and in everything we believe that choosing to follow His guide becomes our new nature. We just do it, not even thinking there is another way. We cannot attempt to live this new life by our own strength; we must accept from Yahweh new hearts and allow Him to make us new people. Our old selves must die, and then we will truly be born all over again.
There is not one thing in all of the Scriptures that He tells us to do that is not for the best. As long as our hearts are pure, our actions will follow, and we will receive His blessings. We are either blessed or cursed. There is no neutrality when it comes to Yahweh's Word. If we live a life of continuous sin, we will be cursed.

This brings us to the next question: what is sin? Again, many people have different ideas of what is good or bad, right or wrong. However, the Scriptures are very clear as to what sin is. Living against Yahweh's commands is sin. This is why we must learn what His Word says — so we can have knowledge of what is most pleasing to Yahweh. Then we must follow it with action.

From a health standpoint, if we are living in sin and know it is wrong, it would be very uncomfortable for us to live each day. Physically, mentally, and spiritually we will be in discomfort. Another word for discomfort is *disease*.

Yahweh does not give us diseases. We inflict ourselves with disease, and Yahweh will either allow it to happen or not to happen; however, He wants us to make the wise choice and to be healthy all the time. He gives us the information to live healthy lives and the freedom to make our own choices.

Yahweh — not a doctor, but the one who created us — knows our bodies better than we do. He is the ultimate doctor, and prayer is the best medicine. If we listen to Him and what He wants us to do, we will be healed.

We must continuously pray to know what Yahweh wants and read Scripture often to confirm that it is of Yahweh. Once we know what Yahweh wants, we must react and do what He tells us to do to experience His blessings.

Your Days Shall Be Many!

Listen, My son, receive what I say, and the years of your life will be many. —Proverbs 4:10

Originally, Yahweh created us to live a very long time, thousands of years at least. Some even say forever. However, the sin of man altered that reality. In the Old Covenant, we see that as sin increased, man's days were shortened. People had been living to nearly a thousand years, but by Noah's day, it was greatly reduced. By Moses' day, it was reduced even more.

The Scriptures clearly show us that it's possible to die before our appointed time.

> *Don't be foolish! Why should you die before your time?*
> —Ecclesiastes 7:17
>
> *Bloodthirsty and deceitful men will not live out half their days.*
> —Psalms 55:23 [NIV]
>
> *The fear of Yahweh adds length to life, but the years of the wicked are cut short.* —Proverbs 10:27

The Scriptures also show us we can add years to our set time. In 2 Kings 20:5, Yahweh healed King Hezekiah. He asked in prayer, and Yahweh added fifteen years to his life. King Hezekiah was on his last breath, but because of his repentance, Yahweh saw his heart and responded.

> *For with Me, your days will be increased; years will be added to your life.* —Proverbs 9:11

The quality of our lives is much more important than the length of our lives. However, if the quality of our lives is filled with joy and good health, and we are in a love affair with Yahweh, we would want to have very long lives. In today's world, people are getting sick and dying at younger and younger ages. The people that are living longer are doing so only with the help of drugs and equipment. If left on their own, they would die much earlier than people of the past.

Not only does the Torah give us an instruction guide of what good and evil are, but Yahweh gives us time to get right with His Word. We have already seen the example of Rahab being spared. During the time of Noah, Yahweh gave the people 120 years to get right with His Word. This 120 years is often seen as the age many can achieve, but Yahweh does not limit our age. He was just telling the people you have 120 years to get right before the flood comes. Many people after the flood lived to over 120.

This is no limit to the age of a righteous person. We all have to die someday, but Yahweh promises those who are righteous will live long lives. Because there are many life-shortening things in our lives today that we may not have control over, such as pollution in the air, etc., these things should not be excuses. These things may shorten our lives by only a few years, but we should still live long lives.

In today's times, most people die before their set times because of their wickedness. We cannot overlook the importance of the Torah. The Torah is Yahweh's guidebook, and all the other books of the Scriptures are given as examples and testimonials of how to understand and apply the Torah guide to our lives. We have many examples in the Scriptures of people who followed that guidebook, and their long lives showed it.

Many Israelites with Moses in the desert committed great sin against Yahweh by rejecting the message Yahweh was giving via Moses. These Israelites brought the sins of Egypt with them when they left and were not willing to let go of them. Yahweh tells us our days should be long and pleasurable. That's for the righteous man. The average age during the time of Moses was between 70 and 80 years old.

> *Seventy years are given to us! Some may even reach eighty.*
> —Psalms 90:10 [NLT]

The average age of man today is even shorter than this. There are more people today living to older ages, but there are also many more people dying at a younger age. The people living at older ages are just barely surviving in old age homes, not enjoying their later years. Moses and many other mighty men of Yahweh were able to hike the desert, climb mountains, and do many other great physical activities in their later years.

If you want to live a long, healthy life, get right with Yahweh's guide, and He will bless you. Sin equals disease, and it is disease that will shorten our lives. Other than an accident not in our control, the Scriptures say disease is unnatural, and we are not supposed to experience it. If we lived disease-free lives, we would be living to an age close to Yahweh's plan, and we would have much vitality and energy.

Emotions vs. Yahweh's Shalom

If we worry as much as the media would like, our emotional health will be at risk of damage. Today, most people live in fear and confusion. We must have control over our emotions to be safe. Losing control of emotions leads to addiction. Addiction to anything is not healthful and can become very harmful. The best way to get control over your emotions is to live as closely as possible to our Creator's guidebook.

In mental disease, there is a lack of emotional control. One of the most harmful influences in the world today leading to negative information overload is watching television. Once considered a luxury, so many people now consider television a necessity. In reality, it's a poison box that relays deadly messages to people every single day in their own homes, draining emotions. Through television, we're programmed by the media to do whatever they want us to do. That's why it's called "programming." Most people who watch television are addicted to it.

Most of the information from TV, radio, newspapers, and so on is extremely destructive and will put anyone's health into a negative state. The main result of today's media impact is to make people worry about everything. Most of the information the media presents, including the way in which it's presented, is slanted toward that end.

One of the problems is that we are trained in today's world, even programmed, to listen to the media, Hollywood, and the popular word on the street. This would be wonderful if all the above were using Yahweh's guidebook as their foundation, but they are not. They're going in the opposite direction. When you listen to the media, you're going further and further away from what Yahweh wants for us. They have taken prayer out of the schools; they're telling us we have no rights and that Yahweh's words are opinion and not fact. Even worse, they have replaced His words with a New Age religion that is false and harmful for us. It is dangerous and evil. To be healthy, we must reverse the tide and go back to what Yahweh wanted for us in all areas of life.

Although many educational shows on television are good for the mind, we are controlled to watch them at certain times instead of when we want. Another problem with TV programs is that the commercial break is so often filled with some form of a negative message.

Once we've chosen our outside influence, the brain carries the message to the rest of the body on a chemical level to our cells, and on an electrical level to the central nervous system. This is why it's so important to make sure the outside influence is not based negatively on worry, but is positive and spiritual.

The next step is for the message to be biologically carried out on a cellular level. Many diseases today, such as cancer, are diseases on a cellular level. Poor diet and other factors can be the cause, but surely this outside influence is of extreme importance. The outside influence we choose must come from the most positive source, Yahweh!

The only answer is either never to watch television, or to watch it only on your own terms with a VCR or DVD player. That's the only way you can be sure to watch what you want when you want. It puts you in control of yourself. When you're programmed, someone else has control over you. Losing your control can be harmful to your health.

But even with VCRs and DVDs, there is still an issue. I didn't understand this until I finally got rid of my television set completely. This truly opened up a whole new freedom in thinking and increased the level of my health. Try it! It might seem hard, but unplug your television set for one month. Put it in the closet, and don't think about it for a month. The first few days will be hard, but when you realize all the extra time you have on your hands, you will wonder why you didn't do that sooner. But be careful! Just one minute of television can drag you back into the downward spiral where television usually leads people.

CHAPTER 7

Knowledge is Key: Listen and Obey. That is the Duty of Every Believer!

> *It is because My people are foolish — they do not know Me; they are stupid children, without understanding, wise when doing evil; but they don't know how to do good.* —Jeremiah 4:22

'Proverb' is another word for 'wisdom.' Wisdom is not a bad thing; in fact, the Scriptures tell us that it is the stability of our lives. The greatest wisdom we can have is the wisdom of Yahweh. The more you know about someone, the more you can discern if you like that person or not. Once you like someone, the more you find out about him, the more you will enjoy his friendship and fall in love with him. Many people who do not read the Scriptures or know Yahweh do not understand the kindness and joy He gives.

Knowledge will strengthen your faith and help make it easier to live a righteous life. We can be seriously misled without good knowledge and true understanding. Many people believe they are doing good and following a good doctrine, but without knowledge, many have been led astray. We simply need knowledge to survive!

> *And to human beings He said, "Look, fear of Yahweh is wisdom! Shunning evil is understanding!"* —Job 28:28

Knowledge of Yahweh comes by having a personal relationship with Him. We can learn even more of how to continuously keep a solid relationship with Him through His Word. His Word confirms who He is, what He wants, and how we can live our lives to please Him.

King Solomon was one of the wisest men ever to live, and he knew the importance of knowledge. When Yahweh told King

Solomon he could have anything he wanted, Solomon's answer pleased Yahweh. Solomon did not ask for gold or silver. He did not ask for fame. He asked for knowledge, not just knowledge, but more wisdom than anyone else.

> *Therefore, give Your servant an understanding heart able to administer justice to Your people, so that I can discern between good and bad.* —1 Kings 3:9

King Solomon asked for understanding to discern good from evil. Many times in Scripture, you can exchange 'sickness' or 'disease' for 'evil', and it would fit perfectly. The opposite of sickness is health, so Solomon is not only asking for understanding about good and evil, but also wisdom to understand health and disease.

Yahweh answered his request and gave him amazing wisdom and knowledge. Also because King Solomon didn't ask for wealth or fame, Yahweh not only blessed him with all he asked for, but also gave him amazing fame and fortune in all things.

It is knowledge that can lead us out of the darkness and into the light. With wisdom and knowledge of why we are sick and diseased, we can understand what we must do to get well again. Knowledge is a powerful tool in the health puzzle of life. However, with great knowledge comes great responsibility. If we don't have new knowledge about something, it is hard to be held accountable for it. This is one reason so many people will harden their hearts and not be open to learning anything new.

I see many people reject the health information I share because they don't want to change their diets. They are so addicted to the foods that they eat. They don't want to hear it is bad for them because once I prove that to them, they know they should change. But because the addiction is so great or eating a certain way for so long is such a comfort zone to them, they choose to keep doing what they are doing, and they continue to suffer for it.

Doing the same things the same way over and over again and expecting different results, they say, is the very definition of insanity! I see many people who get an operation to cut disease out of their bodies, but they continue to live the same way after their operations, creating again the same diseases. You must change your ways if you want the problem to go away and stay away.

In the same manner, there are people who have miraculous healings, but go back to living lives of sin. Their problems that were healed will come back. After Yeshua healed the lame man by the pool (John 5:8), Yeshua said, *"See, you are well! Now stop sinning, or something worse may happen to you!"* (John 5:14).

So lack of knowledge is an issue today when it comes to health and sickness, but once we get that knowledge, we are supposed to put it onto action. Knowledge that is not used wisely is foolishness.

Even if we do not have a clear understanding of what a scripture passage is saying, we are supposed to go way beyond our understanding when reading Scripture and have faith that what it is saying is true and important to follow.

There is so much revealed to us in the Scriptures that can keep us happy and healthy. This is why the Scriptures comprise the best health book ever written. Lack of knowledge — along with rejection of knowledge — can be man's downfall and lead to serious sickness.

> *My people are destroyed from lack of knowledge. Because you have rejected knowledge, I also reject you as My priests; because you have ignored the law of your Creator, I also will ignore your children.*
> —Hosea 4:6 [NIV]

In this verse above, we see how lack and/or rejection of knowledge not only will harm us, but also can harm our children because of our iniquities. We must consciously seek wisdom and knowledge of the Scriptures.

> *He will be the stability of your times, a wealth of salvation, wisdom and knowledge, and fear of Yahweh, which is His treasure.*
> —Isaiah 33:6

Understanding of Yahweh's Word comes to those who are

wise if they put the time into studying His Word. The Scriptures come alive with each word that is read. The more knowledge we have about Yahweh and Yeshua, the clearer the messages of the Scriptures become.

Yahweh will give wisdom to those who ask for it and study the good Word.

> *Many will be purified, made spotless and refined, but the wicked will continue to be wicked. None of the wicked will understand, but those who are wise will understand.* —Daniel 12:10 [NIV]

The Scriptures are not hard to understand; they are historical stories that we can use as lessons and examples of how to live. The Scriptures are to give us knowledge and wisdom. To receive the blessings of a long, healthy, happy, joyous life, the answer is revealed to us in the wisdom of the Scriptures.

> *My son, don't forget My teaching, keep My commands in your heart;*
> *for they will add to you many days, years of life and peace.*
> —Proverbs 3:1-2

This proverb explains how to live a nice, long life in peace and joy: receive My sayings, do not forget My Torah, and guard My commands.

> *Here is what Yahweh says: A curse on the person who trusts in humans, who relies on merely human strength, whose heart turns away from Yahweh.* —Jeremiah 17:5

> *Blessed is the man who trusts in Yahweh; Yahweh will be his security.* —Jeremiah 17:7

Summing up the importance of having knowledge, Yeshua tells us—

> *All the words from My mouth are righteous; nothing false or crooked is in them.*
>
> *They are all clear to those who understand and straightforward to those who gain knowledge.* —Proverbs 8:8-9

How to Gain and Maintain Knowledge of the Scriptures

To gain and maintain knowledge of the Scriptures, we need to—

- Read the Scriptures in order from front to back.
- Study the Scriptures each day, even if only for a few minutes, but aim for at least a half hour or even better, one hour.
- Read different translations to get new insight on the same scriptures.
- Read the study notes that go along with many scriptures.
- Try to spend extra time, question people, or do an internet search if you don't understand a verse.
- Listen to radio and audios often about the Scriptures.
- Download audios on MP3 players, and listen to them while waiting in lines.

PART 2
Diet according to the Scriptures

CHAPTER 8

How We Have Forsaken Yahweh's Diet Plan: Let Each Generation Tell Its Children of Your Mighty Acts.

> *Things which are hidden belong to Yahweh our Creator. But the things that have been revealed belong to us and our children forever, so that we can observe all the words of this Torah.*
> —Deuteronomy 29:29

We have a responsibility as believers to accomplish the goals established during our creation. Yahweh didn't create us to wander around doing little and being lazy. We each have a job and responsibility, and we can only accomplish them to our fullest potential if we abide by Yahweh's guidelines.

On the topic of eating, Yahweh has revealed to us precisely what has been predestined to be our food and a timetable for supreme digestion. He also provided us with a list of acceptable and unacceptable foods. He revealed this so we recognize how to maintain our health and keep our temples (our bodies) pure and clean. This has always been an element of His divine plan. We each have been encoded with the apparatus to carry out all He requests of us.

> *"For I know what plans I have in mind for you," says Yahweh, "plans for well-being, not for bad things; so that you can have hope and a future."* —Jeremiah 29:11

Yahweh will by no means ask us to perform an act that is not achievable. Each deed He requests is for our well-being and is completely capable of being accomplished. The world's pleasures have seduced man away from Yahweh's desires. The enemy influences countless people to avoid Yahweh's eating patterns by way of fear and lack of knowledge. We are called to be doers of the Word and never to stop thinking about the model Yeshua has set for us in His compliance to Torah.

Yahweh provided instructions about all matters of life, including commands concerning eating patterns. He bestowed this eating prototype for our own benefit so we can enjoy long lives (Deuteronomy 4:40, Proverbs 4:10) in peace and comfort.

> *We are Yahweh's masterpiece. He has created us anew in Yeshua, so we can do the good things He planned for us long ago.*
> —Ephesians 2:10 [NLT]

During creation, Yahweh planned for us to perform profitable things. Eating a diet preordained for us by Yahweh is the only option to achieve superior health. Any altered eating plan is not acceptable to Yahweh. People who continue to exist on a separate eating plan are surviving only as a result of His mercy, giving them time to grasp the consequences that result from their actions.

> *For many are invited, but few are chosen* [or choose].
> —Matthew 22:14

We each have a choice to decide and a plan to follow. Our physical health and eternal salvation will be the result. The supreme choice is to acknowledge Yeshua for who He says He is. After that, the upmost decision we are asked to make is to keep the Torah. It is foolish to consider you can recognize Yeshua for who He claims to be and not desire to live in compliance to His instructions and guide. These cannot be separated. One must follow the other. All of the original followers of Yeshua kept the Torah as their upmost guide.

Of all the various topics of discussion, Yahweh's eating patterns seem amongst the most commonly deserted.

This part of the book is about the return to Yahweh's eating plan. I will expose how we have abandoned His methods and how to recapture what was destined to be the standard for each and every one of us. Regardless of the diet you consume at present, you have the capability to return to the diet He has planned and designed for you.

Pertaining to diet, there are three key areas we no longer pay attention to. Each is essential to our health.

1. Give proper consideration to His instructions on acceptable foods.
2. Keep His intended eating timetable.
3. Refuse to make food an idol.

Assemble a strategy to comply with these three matters, and you will transform your health to its peak level while pleasing your Maker in addition. These three matters are the focal point of this part of the book and should educate you in relation to eating according to the Scriptures. In addition to diet, other topics such as water, sleep, fresh air, and exercise are all gifts Yahweh has blessed us with to be healthy.

Yahweh has never altered His set design since the beginning of time. What He intended to be best for us then is still ideal for us today. Man is repeatedly probing a system in opposition to Yahweh's. This pattern started in the Garden of Eden with Adam and Eve and is very common today. People have developed self-destructive behavior in order to appease their fleshly desires.

For instance, when it comes to our food, big businesses are altering and hybridizing seeds, providing us with unreliable carbon copies of Yahweh's healthy seeds. In addition to this disharmonic procedure, the government is passing laws making it difficult for small farmers to stay in business by allowing big corporations exclusive rights to plant seeds that have always been planted for countless years by anyone who chose to do so.

Each dollar spent on food supplied by big corporations takes money away from the small farmer trying to survive. But the small farmer, like the big farmer, is also going against Yahweh's guide, because he has abandoned Yahweh's rule of not letting the land rest every seven years as we are ordered to do in the Scriptures. He is also using hybrid seeds.

As challenging as it may be to obey scripture in our present day, there is no justification not to make your best attempt. Yahweh will never demand us to carry out an act that is unattainable.

The Scriptures proclaim that the commandments will not be burdensome. Yet this is only accurate if our faith is strong and our hearts are completely with Yahweh. If so, your actions and life will be a shining light in this world of darkness.

> *The lamp of your body is the eye. When you have a 'good eye'* [generous spirit], *your whole body is full of light; but when you have an 'evil eye'* [stingy spirit], *your body is full of darkness.* —Luke 11:34

It's simple to make excuses and point blame at others, but have you examined and carried out Yahweh's plan for yourself? Have you been following His eating patterns? Do you seek to purchase unaltered foods?

All this disobedience and rebellion has mystified believers about what commands are supposed to still be kept in our present day. It's a challenging issue that has divided assemblies far and wide. In spite of everything, if a believer is proficient in the study of the Torah, there should be no qualm about the issue.

Nearly everyone who reads the Scriptures nowadays is advised to read only the New Covenant (Testament), though Yeshua and all His original followers daily read the first five books of the Scriptures: Genesis, Exodus, Leviticus, Numbers, and Deuteronomy. The bulk of the teachings of Yeshua, Moses, Paul, and all the prophets were from these five books. They are identified as the Torah. The Torah contains all the instructions about eating according to Yahweh's pattern. It is essential we all gain knowledge of this lesson.

The Scriptures reveal Yahweh's plan in regard to all matters. With proficient investigation, any person can appreciate that Yahweh's eating patterns have not changed over time. Yahweh knew from creation that people's assessments and motives would change, and they would be led away from his instructions. He knew exactly what was going to happen to the food, the people, and the land. He also knew that no matter how hard things seemed, there would always be a few who would seek to keep His Torah (instructions), regardless of what the majority chose.

Daniel is an excellent model of how those who stick to Torah are blessed. Yahweh blessed Daniel with strength, understanding, and great health. Daniel ate according to the instructions found in the Torah. Do you notice the link? Informed that he would be put to death if he refused to eat the foods of the king (that went against the Torah), Daniel kept his faith in Yahweh and rejected any food that was not allowed per Yahweh's instruction guide, and it saved his life.

Ultimately your life is under threat just like Daniel's. It is not the identical set of circumstances, but you will also increase the years of your life by rejecting food Yahweh warned you not to eat. Retain faith no matter the circumstances, and you will be blessed.

Microwaves, frying, and manipulating foods have no role in Yahweh's eating plan. Do not be deceived anymore by marketing and advertising claiming that it is essential to abide by their plan. All your body requires to flourish is within Yahweh's foods.

As we come closer to the return of Yeshua, an increasing number of people are seeking to return to the eating plan designed for our bodies. In all things, people are learning knowledge that was lost but meant to be used. After many years of straying from Yahweh's eating pattern, we may find it difficult to take pleasure in the taste of Yahweh's fresh foods, because our tastebuds have adapted to processed, altered foods. But rest assured that as you return to the original eating plan meant for you, your whole body will again enjoy the foods you have been designed to consume. Your health and energy will be restored, and your entire body will be healthy once more — the way it was always meant to be.

Discontinue transgression of Yahweh's Torah immediately! Don't make foolish statements like, "I will wait until the new year," "I just want to finish what I have in my kitchen cabinets before changing," or "When I get sick, I'll change."

Why wait? Man's ignorance makes him think these foolish statements are wise. On the contrary, they are thoughtless, irrational statements that will do no good.

And idiotic excuses such as, "I don't have money, time, or knowledge to eat healthfully," I hear all the time. Seek His will, and He will provide for you all you need. You cannot believe only half of His Word is true. It's either all true or all false. If you believe Yeshua came to save you from your sins, you must also have faith in Yahweh's eating plan.

The apostle Paul wrote that our bodies are temples of the Set-apart Spirit (1 Cor. 6:19), and it follows that we should care for our bodies as gifts from Yahweh. Eating in the way Yahweh had originally intended for us is one of the countless ways we give thanks to Him for providing us with such superb nourishment.

The Scriptures clearly show us that if we make the wrong choices, we can die before our appointed times. Most so-called believers will agree that suicide is a sin, but they continue to live in a way that is going to end their lives before their appointed times. Whether it takes one quick act or lasts years, knowingly supporting the habits that will end your life prematurely is also suicide. We can do our best to follow the path that Yahweh has chosen and not be led astray by the temptations of this world.

Let's investigate the three common areas of eating the majority of us need to return to.

CHAPTER 9

Nutrition according to the Scriptures: It Is Better to Trust in Yahweh than to Put Confidence in Man.

Then Yahweh said, "Here! Throughout the whole earth I am giving you as food every seed-bearing plant and every tree with seed-bearing fruit." —Genesis 1:29

There are many ideas and concepts regarding nutrition and what foods are most nutritious for the human body. Man has discovered many of these ideas and concepts recently and finds new information as each day passes about nutrition and how it relates to the body. As much as we have discovered, there is still a great deal undiscovered. Since we don't have all the facts about nutrients and how our bodies respond to them, wouldn't it make sense to pay attention to the designer of the nutrients and the Maker of the body they go into? Only this will assure we are eating the finest foods in the best way possible.

It was our Creator Yahweh who first separated the saltwater from the fresh, made dry land, and planted a garden. He even made animals and fish before making one human being. He made what we needed before we were even born. If He designed our bodies and knows every single hair on our heads, I'm sure He knows what we should eat and when we should eat it.

Not all nutrients have the same effect, and ignoring His plan can be dangerous, even fatal. Take herbs for example. There is no doubt that herbs can be very healing to the body, but taken in excess can result in a toxic situation. Furthermore, poisonous herbs taken in just a minute quantity can have grave consequences. So we must be careful to give our bodies precisely what will benefit them; anything else will contribute to disease.

Can you identify every plant, herb, flower, grain, nut, and seed?

Each has an entirely distinctive uniqueness that can be beneficial to various organs of the body. I come across countless people that advocate one food for "healing" or one food for "health" that is preeminent for everyone. However, the body is so complex, and there are loads of variables to contemplate, that one food cannot "cure all." Also, another thing to ponder is that eating nourishing food will help preserve excellent health, but what fare should be taken during situations of disease? When a health issue takes place, how do you discern the perfect foods for the situation?

Our magnificent Creator provides us with all our needs. In His own way, He reveals to us the signs we need to unlock the mystery of each plant to discover its medicinal properties. Long ago, primitive cultures were proficient in use of all the plants and herbs, as they were preordained to be food, medicine, and even construction material.

The Scriptures are like a treasure map guiding us to the solutions and to questions that man has not yet figured out. If we give prudent awareness to His words, we can gain hidden knowledge about nutrition that will transform the way we live. Yahweh reveals to us what foods are toxic and nontoxic. He also enlightens us to comprehend how much is adequate for our requirements. He even makes us aware of the best places and times to consume our meals. Beyond doubt, one of the most exceptional discoveries has been the discovery of nutrients in certain foods and how they affect each organ of the body.

There is a saying, "Let food be your medicine." I'm not convinced lots of people heard it, because it appears food has turned into their poison. Nevertheless, Yahweh didn't plan that to be the situation. Countless people nowadays have abused the magnificent gift He has given us as nourishment and twisted it into a deadly weapon. We all die and leave our physical body at some point, but He never designed for us to pass away as a consequence of overindulgence in food. Our bodies were not fashioned to consume loads of candy, cakes, cookies, and processed foods. We were designed to enjoy the fruits and vegetables existing in the Garden of Eden, and even them in small amounts.

All fruits and vegetables have been given to us to sustain and heal our bodies. Here are various common foods and how they heal our bodies:

Carrots — Carrots are good for the eyes because they contain nutrients that support good eyesight and greatly enhance blood flow to and from the eyes. Fittingly, if you slice a carrot, the cross section looks like the human eye.
Tomatoes — Most red vegetables are good for the blood, but the tomato when sliced has four chambers just like the heart, the organ of the body that pumps blood. Research shows tomatoes are loaded with lycopene and are indeed pure heart and blood food.
Grapes — Grapes are another excellent food for the heart. If you look at clusters of grapes, they usually hang in the shape of hearts. Each grape is like a blood cell, vitalizing the blood of the body.
Walnuts — Walnuts have folds that look very similar to the brain. The oils found in walnuts are excellent for the brain.
Celery — Celery comes in the shape of bones. The minerals in celery are excellent for good bone support.
Avocados — Avocados are a true super food, especially for the health and function of the womb and cervix of the female. If you look at a sliced avocado, it is in the shape of these organs.
Figs — Figs are a wonderful food. Figs have been discovered to increase the motility of male sperm. Interestingly, they have many seeds and hang in twos when they grow.

As you can observe, Yahweh does not compose things too complicated to understand. The dilemma is that nearly everyone is hurrying through life, never taking the time to examine all the beauty He has created. One person may just see an orange as a round object when others see it as a gift from Yahweh that is stunning to the eye, sweet in taste, and with a brilliant odor.
As you observe your food, you appreciate that you do not have to be a scientist to know what food does for every part of the body. Until additional information is revealed to us, we ought to

stay away from new, processed foods we are not familiar with and place our reliance on what is established.

The enemy is extremely clever in deceiving the unstable believer. He tricks people by convincing them there is no link between diet and health. If you want to change results, you must change the action. If your health suffers as a result of your diet, the answer doesn't remain in doctors or drugs; on the contrary, it remains in Yeshua.

The ordinary person nowadays eats too many foods containing processed sugar, high fat, animal proteins, and an insufficient quantity of fresh fruits, vegetables, nuts, and seeds. Others who believe a vegetarian diet is most beneficial often persist in consuming an excess of fat, sugar, and protein from vegetarian junk foods, and in spite of everything, still not enough fresh foods; so they suffer from the same illnesses. Finally, they throw in the towel and exclaim there is no link between health and diet. So they go back to where they started.

Few people will ultimately realize there is a link between diet and health. However, in spite of everything they have learned, they will unwisely carry on their uncontrollable desire to satisfy their tastebuds and full stomachs.

If you want to get well, you can't change only the name of the diet and anticipate recovery. Replacing one unhealthful way of eating with another is not going to succeed.

It's time you start the ball rolling. Begin eating according to the Scriptures. A tremendous first step would be to eliminate all processed foods. Anything that comes in a bag, container, box, can, or bottle is not ideal for your body, especially if it doesn't have an expiration date on the package. Do not be fooled by marketing words and advertisements. The skin of the fruit or vegetable is the finest packaging. Yahweh didn't make mistakes. He intended produce to grow in every climate. Everything we require is found in a wide variety of fruits, vegetables, nuts, seeds, and unprocessed animal products.

CHAPTER 10

Yahweh's Designed Eating Plan: May Your Eyes Take Delight in Following His Ways.

Fools! Didn't the One who made the outside make the inside too?
—Luke 11:40

Loads of people today are searching to find the supreme diet, one that will give them ultimate energy, keep off weight, and combat disease. Due to this popular demand, countless marketers are pushing all types of diet plans merely for profit. Few provide the answers people are seeking. The good news is that the search has led people to the Scriptures to inquire about the diet of the Bible. People are probing the Scriptures now more than ever before.

The Scriptures reveal a great deal about the ultimate diet we should eat. Countless passages in the Scriptures precisely relate to diet and food. Some more well-known examples are Genesis 1:29, Genesis 9:3, Leviticus 11, and Daniel 1. However, not all scriptures that mention food are about diet. There are numerous verses and parables given that mention a particular way of eating that actually do not concern food, but instead are used metaphorically.

With good study, the diet plan our Creator designed us to eat will reveal itself. Still, there is great controversy amongst Bible students about the genuine diet of the Scriptures. Some people believe it doesn't matter what we eat so long as we bless it. However this is not true. Yahweh alerted us to what foods are best and what foods are harmful so we can maintain our health.

Of all the discussions about the diet of the Scriptures, the vegetarian vs. animal-eating debate leads the way. But even amongst meat eaters, there is a disagreement about which meats can be eaten and which shouldn't. The Scriptures are clear about all these topics. Any disagreement is not due to lack of information. Everything we need to know about diet is found in the Scriptures. Sometimes it may seem the Scriptures contradict the message, but it's only our lack of understanding that keeps us on both sides of the issue.

Anyone with good knowledge of the all the scriptures from Genesis to Revelation should agree that it's very clear what the Scriptures say about the diet issue. The reason you don't find many people who agree on the topic is because most people have not read all the scriptures even once, yet alone studied the issue. A person needs to read the Scriptures several times before getting a clear understanding.

On the topic of eating, other than what the Scriptures reveal, we also have to take into consideration other factors in order to come up with the answer for what is best for us today. There is a big decline in the quality of food today because man continues to look for profit and greed and not at our health needs. Just about every food source Yahweh gave us, from the crops to the animals, is not as clean and nutritious as Yahweh meant it to be. We have to be very wise to understand His exact plan and how we can come close to achieving it today.

Another factor is that just because it is not written in Scripture doesn't mean it's not an issue. Yahweh intended us to always seek to give our bodies the best possible nourishment at the best possible times. Eating from a microwave oven or eating a highly processed food that comes in a box is not taking care of our bodies as well as possible.

Another thing to consider about eating according to the Scriptures is that the Scriptures say everything that comes from Yahweh is good, but they don't say everything that comes from Yahweh is good for us to eat. Yahweh has a reason for everything He created. He created us to live a certain way and supplied us with the information and wisdom to figure out what is good and what is not good for our bodies.

The bottom line comes down to the fact that Yahweh never wanted us to defile our temples (our bodies). Whether by poison chemicals on our produce or toxic drugs in the animals, these all defile the body and are not what Yahweh wanted.

Daniel is a great example of having to choose between going against Yahweh to please man or going against man's ways to please Yahweh.

It was a very easy decision for him to make. Daniel always chose the side of Yahweh, no matter what the consequences. Daniel was told if he didn't bow down to pagan gods, he would be killed. But Daniel had no fear and stayed strong. He picked faithfulness over emotion.

There is another passage, Daniel 1:14, that confirms many things when it comes to diet and health, as well as sticking to Yahweh's Torah regardless of the pressure. No matter how much pressure from the world, Daniel rejected the king's diet and said, "I will only stick to Yahweh's diet," and he was blessed for it with the best health, as seen in Daniel 1:11-20.

After only ten days of eating according to Yahweh's diet plan, Daniel and his three friends had ten times more beauty, knowledge, and wisdom than any of the other slaves. They were in a very stressful environment but didn't resort to emotional eating on junk food, as so many people do today while blaming it on their circumstances.

Listening to Yahweh's guide is not only scriptural, but is also a must if we want to regain our health and keep it. We must listen to Yahweh's guide and stick with it no matter what.

Why don't you give it a try? For one month, try eating 100% according to Yahweh's diet plan, avoiding all the junk foods and unclean meats that go against his plan, and realize the great results. Once you see how much better you feel, you should become convinced.

Seek Yahweh while He is available, call on Him while He is still nearby. —Isaiah 55:6

Yahweh's Eating Plan

Amongst all the different diets and ways to eat in today's

world, no matter how often or how much the idea of a healthy diet might change according to what's popular in the world, the diet and health principles of Yahweh never change and always work. Unfortunately, people are choosing the world's diet over Yahweh's diet.

As we look at the diet choices people have made and the suffering they experience for it, we can identify the areas people must repent of and correct if they want to experience the full blessing of health that Yahweh has to offer.

How did Yahweh plan for us to take care of our temples?

Man was a vegetarian in the Garden of Eden at the beginning of time. After Adam sinned, man was kicked out of the Garden of Eden and had to find a new way to survive. He now had to work for his food. He was either planting or hunting. Even though it doesn't say man ate meat or started to consume animal products such as milk and eggs at that time, Abel became a shepherd (Genesis 4:2), so there is a good hint that man was no longer a strict vegan as was such in the Garden of Eden. One question up for debate is whether man was consuming animal flesh at that point or just consuming milk, butter, and eggs but no flesh?

If Abel was consuming meat or other animal products, then he must have chosen a way to survive that went against Yahweh's original instructions that fruits and vegetables are the food for man (Genesis 1:29). According to the timing in scripture, Yahweh had not yet given man permission to eat animals. It was nevertheless in Yahweh's divine plan for the death of animals to take place.

Another possibility is that Abel was still a vegan, but he became a shepherd because he was concerned with having the best possible sacrifices to offer Yahweh. Abel knew blood had to be shed to please Yahweh.

Yahweh himself set this example by providing the first coverings for Adam and Eve through the sacrifice of animals. No sooner had they fallen than Yahweh intervened and made coats of skins to clothe them. So Yahweh Himself was the first to shed blood to cover man's sin. He set an example for Abel and also gave a view of what was to come by the blood of Yeshua covering all our sins.

> *In fact, according to the Torah, almost everything is purified with blood; indeed, without the shedding of blood, there is no forgiveness of sins.* —Hebrews 9:22

There was no need for animal sacrifices in the Garden originally because there was no sin, but once sin entered, Yahweh provided one of His first lessons for man: the shedding of blood must take place for mercy and forgiveness.

In the Bible, nearly everything is purified with blood. Blood must be shed for remission. You may say blood is repulsive, hateful. Some women faint at the sight of blood, but by blood was the way Yahweh marked out for coming to Him from the very first. Abel came by that way and was accepted. This shows how wicked man's mind and actions of sin are that Yahweh has to go to such an extreme to wake us up.

Still, Yahweh did not yet reveal up to this point what animals were clean or unclean for an offering. Somehow, Able knew how to please Yahweh. A consideration is that Yahweh did reveal to Cain and Able the full instructions for offerings. Abel was obedient and Cain was not.

If Abel did in fact switch to eating animals without Yahweh's permission, Yahweh showed His amazing mercy towards the disobedience to His instructions when He accepted Abel's animal sacrifice. Just like today, if we come to Him with our best sacrifice and a sincere heart, He will always show us His mercy. On the other hand, if we follow His instructions but fail to offer Him our best sacrifice (Genesis 4:3), such as Cain did, we will not be accepted. What would be best is obeying His instructions and giving him our best sacrifice with a sincere heart.

Sixteen hundred years later, Yahweh saved Noah via the ark. When Noah left it, he offered the blood of every clean beast and fowl on the altar. The second dispensation was founded on blood; it came between Noah and man's sin. The world was set up afresh under Noah, but it began from the blood.

The Scriptures neither record nor show Yahweh explaining to Noah until after the flood what animals were approved for offerings. Yet He instructs Noah to take seven pairs of approved animals and only one pair of unapproved. How would Noah know? Yahweh must have revealed the information to Noah somehow, even though those instructions are not recorded in Scripture until the time of Moses.

There are no precise answers to what the diet was once man left the garden and before the great flood that washed away the evil people of the earth. Did man eat flesh? If so, did Yahweh allow it?

However, we do know that the death of animals took place, and it was fine with Yahweh because it was all part of His divine plan leading up to the death by bloodshed of Yeshua. And we also know that Yahweh clearly revealed after the flood that we could eat animals.

There was only one restriction given at that time, and it was to be careful not to eat the blood. Consuming the blood was the only restriction because it is the set-apart liquid of life that belongs to Yahweh and should have always been offered to Him. The other restrictions and rules about clean and unclean animals were not recorded until many years afterwards (Leviticus 11 and Deuteronomy 14).

One more interesting fact to consider is that after the flood, Yahweh said that "all animals" were okay to consume as long as no blood was consumed. There were still no instructions for clean or unclean animals. Man's lifespan declined rapidly from the time after the flood to the exodus from Egypt.

Lifespans stopped declining after the instructions for clean and unclean animals were given to Moses. Those who obeyed the instructions regarding clean and unclean animals lived good long lives. However, the lifespans of those who continued to eat unclean animal meat and reject other parts of the Torah continued to decline.

Even though we were given permission to consume animals, Yahweh still showed us His mercy. His instructions not to include unclean animals or the certain fat or blood of animals constituted sort of His rescue plan, or His instructions on how not to suffer while including the animal flesh as part of the diet.

It is significant to note that meat-eating animals are most often the animals Yahweh considers unclean food and instructs us never to eat, while strictly vegetarian animals are mostly approved as clean. The further we progress from getting our nutrients directly from the plants or fruits, the worse our health seems to have gotten.

Yahweh has built our bodies so wonderful and amazing that we can consume certain animals as food and still thrive in health if done with wisdom. We just have to listen and obey. Yet man could not obey those two orders.

The rules given with the permission to consume animal food are (a) do not eat unclean animals, (b) do not eat animals sacrificed to idols, and (c) do not eat the blood or certain fat of the animals. All of these instructions are being ignored today, and we are paying for it with our lack of health.

Just because Yahweh gave man permission to eat meat doesn't mean it had to be added to the diet. There is only one time in the Scriptures man is commanded to eat meat: at Passover. There is some debate about this today. Some quote the Scriptures and say this commandment was giving to us to keep all our generations, while others argue Yeshua was our final sacrifice, so we no longer need to sacrifice and consume a lamb for Passover.

It is important to mention that Paul was a strict keeper of the Torah. Even after his meeting with Yeshua, this did not change. Man's lustful nature has twisted many of the verses and ideas of Paul to make it appear he was saying all animal flesh was okay to consume after the sacrifice of Yeshua. This is not true.

Paul and all the followers of Yeshua and Yeshua himself *never even considered* eating unclean animal flesh. It was so unthinkable when Yahweh told Peter to kill and eat unclean animals. Peter said he never had because he didn't want to defile himself. Yahweh's permission to Peter to eat unclean animals in no way meant it was now okay. He was proving a point to Peter that all believers can be saved by the blood of Yeshua, not only the Jewish people.

Eating unclean animals is, and will always be, a sin according to Scripture. If you are truly born again, you should shudder even at the thought of putting an unclean animal to your lips. Yahweh says we are not even to touch the carcass of an unclean animal, let alone consume it.

If you choose to consume animal flesh or products, that's fine according to the Scriptures, as long as you follow the guidelines. If not, you are committing an abomination to Yahweh and your own temple (body). If a vegan diet is your choice, make sure you get all the protein and other nutrients you need by consuming a good variety of high-quality fruits, vegetables, nuts, and seeds according to Yahweh's schedule, adding supplementation if necessary.

Why would Yahweh change His original plan and now allow meat as part of the diet?

Yahweh didn't change His plan. He never changes! He is always the same yesterday, today, and tomorrow. Since Yahweh never changes, animal consumption would have been part of His original plan. He had just not revealed it to man yet in the Garden. He knew man would disobey His instructions by sinning and be kicked out of the Garden. He also knew man was going to consume meat. We must not view this as a new or improved diet, but part of Yahweh's predesigned divine diet later revealed to us.

In the Scriptures, it says when we are ready, more will be revealed (Luke 8:10). Remember, Yahweh told Noah to take more clean animals than unclean animals into the ark. Seven pairs of clean animals versus one pair of unclean. Yahweh was doing His part in providing us with more clean animals for our sacrifices, but also our food if we chose to eat meat. He knew beforehand many people would make the choice to consume animal flesh. It was all part of his divine plan.

The Scriptures contain several examples concerning various topics that illustrate what was allowed versus what was the true will of Yahweh. They were not always the same. Besides the diet debate, other matters included divorce and polygamy, for example. Each time people chose the nonideal path of appeasing their lust, hardship came along with it. I mention these other topics to show there is a pattern in the Scriptures.

- Yahweh says one thing, but it's men's sinful natures to want something else.
- Yahweh grants them their requests and leaves them to suffer the consequences of their lust.

Yeshua puts this pattern in good perspective when questioned about divorce by the Pharisees. In Matthew 19:8, He says, "Moses permitted divorce only as a concession to your hard hearts, but it was not what Yahweh had originally intended."

Finally the last part of this pattern is where we see Yahweh's wonderful mercy if people repent:

> *There were foolish people who suffered affliction because of their crimes and sins;*
>
> *they couldn't stand to eat anything; they were near the gates of death.*
>
> *In their trouble, they cried to Yahweh, and He rescued them from their distress;*
>
> *He sent His Word and healed them; He delivered them from destruction.* —Psalms 107:17-20

Hopefully, people learn from their poor choices. The above verse claims that if people truly repent, they can reverse the hardships that come along with their unwise decisions. True repentance can only happen if one accepts the blood of Yeshua. Then it must be followed by action. A person cannot make a claim and mean it if the actions do not change. The actions reveal the heart!

CHAPTER 11

Yahweh Said Don't Touch That! A Person without Self-Control Is Like a City with Broken-down Walls!

The earth suffers for the sins of its people, for they have twisted Yahweh's instructions, violated His laws and broken His everlasting covenant. —Isaiah 24:5 [NLT]

Health doesn't begin with what we add to our diet, but what we avoid. The first step in getting back to Yahweh's diet plan is to avoid, or at least cut back on, the foods that were never meant to be consumed in the first place. The enemy is very clever and will tempt you any way he can to live in disobedience to Yahweh. Diet is often the path that leads many people to sin.

The following is a list of foods that we should never consume, starting with the worst and ending with those unhealthful foods that we should at least limit. Still, it is more healthful and suggested to avoid all of these foods. Just because you don't feel ill after consuming them doesn't mean they are not harmful to you. It has been proven that physically, mentally, and spiritually they shorten the quality and quantity of life.

I will first give the complete list, and then we will take a look at each one:

- Unclean animals
- The fat of an animal
- The blood of an animal
- Animals sacrificed to idols
- Animals that have been drugged
- Poison and toxic plans
- Chemical-laden foods
- Hybridized foods
- Processed foods

> *Obey and pay attention to everything I am ordering you to do, so that things will go well with you and with your descendants after you forever, as you do what Yahweh sees as good and right.*
> —Deuteronomy 12:28

Yahweh is our Creator and created all things with a purpose. He has a plan for each thing He created and designed. When we reject that plan, we claim we know better than He did. Many Christians proclaim with their words they want to follow Yahweh's way, but their actions reveal the opposite. They only seem to follow Yahweh when it is pleasing to their flesh. With any sign of discomfort, most people run in the other direction.

In the Scriptures, followers of Yahweh put their lives on the line for Him. Most people today are not even willing give up their comforts and luxuries for Him. The decline in passion to fulfill His commands is a reality that can't be ignored. We live during a time when more people ignore Yahweh's warnings about what is not right to eat and suffer as a result of not being obedient to His instructions. Sickness and disease are prevalent in every nation, but the only times they become issues amongst believers is when disobedience is taking place.

> *Do not depend on your own understanding.*
>
> *Seek His will in all you do, and He will direct your paths.*
> —Proverbs 3:5-6 [NLT]

Do not let your flesh control your actions or create your desires. We cannot pick and choose by what our flesh tells us is best. If you want to be healthy, obey Yahweh's Word, even if it doesn't seem right to you at the time. We need to trust and go on faith that He knows and wants what is best for us. We need to trust him with our whole hearts and let our actions follow.

Unclean Animals

> *You must not eat any detestable animals that are ceremonially unclean.* —Deuteronomy 14:3 [NLT]

Yahweh warned us thousands of years ago that unclean animals are harmful to our health and should never be consumed. Some people claim the dietary rules given to the Hebrews in the Bible do not pertain to them. Science confirms every guideline Yahweh gave in the Torah about eating will benefit all of humankind, regardless of whether they are Hebrew or not.

Yahweh planned for these animals never to be consumed. Even the smallest amounts can be harmful to your health. The following is a partial list. It is not limited to the animals on the list. Exactly which types of animals are unclean are found in the provided scriptures for each listing. To determine if an animal is clean or unclean, compare them to the instructions found in the Scriptures.

Unclean Land Animals

You may not, however, eat the animals named here because they either have split hooves or chew the cud, but not both.
—Leviticus 11:4 [NLT]

Pig (pork), rabbit, raccoon, squirrel, monkey, dog, coyote, fox, wolf, lion, tiger, horse, mule, zebra, bear, camel, elephant, llama, hippo, kangaroo.

Unclean Marine Animals

You may not, however, eat marine animals that do not have both fins and scales. —Leviticus 11:10 [NLT]

Catfish, eel, marlin, shark, abalone, clam, crab, crayfish, lobster, oyster, shrimp, scallops, jellyfish, squid, dolphin, seal, whale.

Unclean Birds

These are the birds you must never eat because they are detestable for you. —Leviticus 11:13 [NLT]

Bat, eagle, osprey, raven, duck, swan, vulture.

Unclean Insects, Rodents, and Other Animals

The Scriptures even give a list of insects and other rodents that should never be consumed in Leviticus 11:20-31. Some of these include frog, toad, crocodile, lizard, snake, turtle, salamander, newt, snail.

Not only does Yahweh warn us to never consume any of the above-mentioned animals, but He also states that they are so harmful to us that we should not even touch their carcasses. From a hygienic standpoint, it has been confirmed that coming into contact with the flesh of these animals often spreads communicable diseases and other harmful germs. Yahweh gave these special instructions to everyone. The ones who obeyed were blessed with good health and long lives.

I find it very interesting that the differences between clean and unclean animals appear to be related to their primary food sources and to their digestive systems. Scavengers that eat anything and everything are not suitable for food, according to Yahweh. Most animals described as clean, and therefore good for food, primarily eat grasses and grains. There are some exceptions to this, such as horses. They eat grasses and are not scavengers, but the Scriptures instruct us that they are not to be eaten because they do not have split hooves. Just as another example of how far we have transgressed, horsemeat, usually considered unthinkable to consume here in the U.S., has recently become very popular due to its lean, tender meat. However, new studies reveal that although horsemeat is considered among the leanest and best meats around the world, it commonly contains viruses and parasites. We again see Yahweh's warning there to help us.

Of all the foods that the Scriptures suggest we should avoid, the sternest warning comes with unclean animals. Ignoring these guidelines causes bad health and violent thinking. According to Scripture, it completely defiles a person for a certain amount of time, making that person ceremonially unclean. This means these people were sent away from everyone else for a certain amount of time (usually till evening) before they could be clean again and return, perhaps to be alone to focus on the abomination they had committed to Yahweh and their own bodies.

Today we do not need to give offerings of animal sacrifices to Yahweh (thanks to the blood of Yeshua); however, Yahweh says we are never to consume any of these animals. If we do, we will also be separated from communion with Yahweh for a certain amount of time until we repent.

Some people may say that this is a ridiculous statement, that Yahweh doesn't care what we consume, and that it will certainly not separate us from Him. It is wicked to believe Yahweh gave us guidelines but doesn't expect us to follow them. He gave these orders to all of our generations for a reason, and Yahweh is far from the wicked (Proverbs 15:29).

Eat No Animal Fat

Say to the people of Israel, "You are not to eat the fat of bulls, sheep or goats.

The fat of animals that die of themselves or are killed by wild animals may be used for any other purpose, but under no circumstances are you to eat it." —Leviticus 7:23-24

Certain fats are healthful, and some very unhealthful. Science recently has identified the fats that benefit us that we need to thrive, while confirming what fats should never be consumed. The amazing thing is the fatty foods that science today says are unhealthful are what Yahweh revealed to us in His Scriptures thousands of years ago that we should never eat. This is not a case of Yahweh catching up with science, but it's the other way around.

There is still so much man has yet to discover for our health, but anyone who has studied the Scriptures can have certain knowledge long before science reveals what is unhealthful. Today, Yahweh and science both agree the fats found in plants and fruits are fats that are important for our health, but certain fats that come from animal flesh are very harmful to our health.

Many fats when cooked are unhealthful! The fats from fruits and vegetables are often consumed uncooked, but animal fat is usually cooked. Cooking the flesh of the animal is the only way to make sure you kill all of the germs and harmful bacteria, but cooking it away from Yahweh's instructions makes the fats even more harmful. Your body uses a tremendous amount of energy trying to digest the prohibited fat of the animal. This cooked animal fat can contribute to clogged arteries, obesity, and a host of other serious health issues. The best answer is to completely avoid the fats of the animal flesh that Yahweh warned not to consume and eat raw fruits and vegetables, nuts, and seeds that contain the good fats.

It is almost impossible to consume animal flesh and not eat some of the fat, because the fat is within the animal flesh that we cannot see and cut away or avoid when eating. Yahweh knows what fats are healthy and harmful and guides us not to avoid all fat but certain fats (Exodus 29:13, Exodus 29:22).

There are certain fatty foods from animals that if raw are healthful and can be consumed in small amounts, such as eggs, milk, cheese, and even fish oil. I believe Yahweh wasn't warning us not to eat these types of fats. It was only certain fat of the flesh that is harmful. The fat found in eggs, milk, cheese, and fish oil from animals raised in healthy environments with clean food sources, and that has not been processed, heated, drugged, or contaminated can be very beneficial to our health.

Some people may be concerned about consuming raw eggs or raw dairy, but there should be more of a concern in cooking these products, as the healthful fat turns to a harmful fat when consumed. Studies show there is very little chance of having any issues if the raw eggs or dairy is organic, free of any drugs, and comes from grass-fed animals.

Eggs, dairy, and fish were common foods consumed by people of the Scriptures. This could be due to the fact they lived in a desert, and this was all that was available to certain people. However, these foods are excellent survival foods when one cannot attain fresher, more healthful food sources, such as a good variety of fruits and vegetables. Today we are in a similar time because big businesses have replaced the small farmer. Our produce is no longer as fresh and healthful as it once was. In certain cases, just like survival times, these foods may help us survive.

I know certain vegetarians who say they would never consume milk, eggs, or fish. I understand their thinking, but being close-minded can led to health issues. We have to take into consideration all the factors in order to decide what the ideal diet is for each of us. With that in mind, we always need to consider Yahweh's guide whenever making choices about our diet.

There is a difference between certain fats found in animal flesh Yahweh instructed us to avoid versus the fat of milk, cheese, and eggs. The fat of fish, one of the most consumed foods in the Scriptures, is not as harmful as that of land animals or birds. According to recent studies, as long as the fish is on Yahweh's approved list and from clean water and prepared the right way, there are some very beneficial fats within those fish.

The problem nowadays is that many of the oceans around the world are polluted, so we must be careful if we choose to eat fish. Some people take cod liver oil to get these healthful fats, but much of the bottling and storage often causes these oils to go rancid. If you do choose this oil, make sure the bottle has an expiration date and is from a reliable source.

I do not recommend eating fish raw because of parasites and other bacteria. However, since Yeshua was seen cooking fish, I will assume the fatty oils in the fish are not affected the same way as the fats in the land animals; so it would be okay to consume cooked fish. But realize that the fish Yeshua was cooking and all the fish consumed back then was wild from the ocean.

Today there are fish farms raising fish. Even if these fish species are on Yahweh's clean list, they should be avoided because of the toxic food and drugs the farms raise these fish on. Studies show the good fat of the clean ocean fish has the correct balance of omega-3 and omega-6 fats, but that is not the same with farm-raised fish that contain an unhealthful balance. So farm-raised fish should be avoided.

Eat No Blood

But you must never eat animals that still have their lifeblood in them. —Genesis 9:4 [NLT]

Blood represents life in Yahweh's divine plan.

For the life of a creature is in the blood. —Leviticus 17:11

Blood represents life in the current body, as well as the blood of Yeshua, meaning the eternal life after we leave our bodies. Life cannot exist without blood.

Blood is never an easy topic to discuss, but it must be spoken about if you want to understand the Scriptures and what they have to say about diet and everything else. In fact, if you are truly a believer and understand Scripture, you cannot avoid the subject, because blood runs throughout the whole Bible. Any religion that is not founded on "the blood" comes from the pit of hell. There is no other foundation. Any other way is not Yahweh's way. All who think they do not need the blood of Yeshua are not saved!

> *For the life of a creature is in the blood, and I have given it to you on the altar to make atonement for yourselves; for it is the blood that makes atonement because of the life.*
>
> *This is why I told the people of Israel, "None of you is to eat blood, nor is any foreigner living with you to eat blood."* —Leviticus 17:11-12

Food with no blood is considered kosher food. When we hear about eating kosher, there are two types of kosher. There is kosher according to the Rabbis, which is more a tradition of man not found in the Scriptures. Then there is kosher according to the written Word from Yahweh. There are several differences between the two, but one of the things they definitely have in common is that the blood of an animal should never be consumed.

When we consume the blood of an animal, we are taking what belongs to Yahweh. Blood sprinkled on the altar during the animal sacrifices represented a foreshadowing of Messiah's blood that would be shed for our sins. Since Yeshua was our final sacrifice, Yahweh no longer requires the blood of the animals to cover our sins. However, this is still a special life-giving liquid that sustains our lives if we keep our bloodstreams clean, uncontaminated by the blood of another animal.

Yahweh designed each one of us with our own individual chemical makeup. If we mix someone else's blood with our own, it can poison our body. Today, doctors can run tests to confirm what blood is safe to mix and what blood is not during an emergency such as a blood transfusion. However, no one ever runs tests on animal blood to see if it is safe to be consumed. Other than mixing of blood by injection, consuming or even touching blood, though not as common as mixing, can also transfer many viruses that can lead to disease and even death.

Blood gives us life, but unhealthy blood can also take it away. One more great example of blood's giving life in Yahweh's divine plan is when He commanded His chosen people on the night of the Passover in Egypt to put blood on their doorposts to cover their houses so no death would enter during the Passover. They were saved when they obeyed. The consequences of disobeying that order from Yahweh would have surely led to the death of the firstborn male in the house. Yahweh's instructions should not be taken lightly.

We are told in the Scriptures to avoid consuming the blood of the animals! This is an overlooked commandment that can have very harmful consequences on your health. Blood carries oxygen and many other elements to prolong life, but blood may also contain viruses and other elements to cause death.

> *Just take care not to eat the blood, for the blood is the life, and you are not to eat the life with the meat.* —Deuteronomy 12:23

In Deuteronomy 12:16, we are commanded to give the blood back to Yahweh via pouring it on the ground like water. Just as Yahweh says, man comes from the dust of the earth and he shall go back to the dust of the earth; so shall the blood of man and animals.

> *Just take care not to eat the blood, for the blood is the life, and you are not to eat the life with the meat.*
>
> *Don't eat it, but pour it out on the ground like water.*
>
> *Do not eat it, so that things will go well with you and with your children after you, as you do what Yahweh sees as right.*
> —Deuteronomy 12:23-25

Animals Sacrificed to Idols

Do not worship Yahweh your Creator in the way these pagan peoples worship their gods.

Rather, you must seek Yahweh your Creator at the place He Himself will choose from among all the tribes for His name to be honored.

There you will bring to Yahweh your burnt offerings, your sacrifices, your tithes, your special gifts, your offerings to fulfill a vow, your freewill offerings, and your offerings of the firstborn animals of your flocks and herds.

There you and your families will feast in the presence of Yahweh your Creator, and you will rejoice in all you have accomplished because Yahweh your Creator has blessed you.
—Deuteronomy 12:4-7 [NLT]

We are warned in the Scriptures not to consume any animal flesh that has been sacrificed to an idol. When was the last time you checked, before sitting down to consume a steak or chicken, where it came from and how it was prepared? It would surely be an odd question to ask the waiter in a restaurant, and I'm sure he wouldn't know the answer. Man was told certain meat can be eaten, but certain meat should never be consumed. There is a conundrum asking if a tree falls in the woods, but no one is there to hear it, does it make a sound? Of course it does. Well, if an animal has been sacrificed to an idol, but you don't know about it, was it still sacrificed to an idol?

There are many idols in today's world — money, cars, etc. — but we have to be careful not to get carried away with this while understanding the dangers of consuming meat or even vegetables offered to other gods. Anything that has been offered as a sacrifice to another god was considered unholy to Yahweh.

In Acts 10:14, Peter says he has never eaten an animal that was defiled and unclean. Unclean can mean an animal that was not on Yahweh's clean list of animals to consume, but defiled surely meant an animal that was offered to another god.

During the times of the Scriptures and even today, there are many so-called gods of this world, but there is only one true Creator. Not only were animals sacrificed to other gods in the

Scriptures, but even children were. Today, I walk into some stores and see statues of images on the floor or certain pictures on the walls that people bow down to and worship. We cannot know for sure how the food is prepared, but if you see these things where you buy your food or where you eat, you should be careful. It is very likely what you are eating has been offered to an idol first.

> *Do not bring any detestable objects into your home, for then you will be destroyed just like them. You must utterly detest such things, for they are set apart for destruction.* —Deuteronomy 7:26 [NLT]

Any item that is detestable to Yahweh should also be detestable to you. Today, people buy and put statues of ancient gods and pictures of cult leaders in their homes and call it art. Everything in your home should reflect praise and love towards Yahweh only and no other gods. This also includes obeying his instructions about eating. Before bringing any food in your home, do some research about its source.

Animals That Have Been Drugged

Hopefully by now you see that Yahweh planned a specially designed diet for all humankind. Still, people's habits and addictions will control them to continue to transgress away from Yahweh's plan. In a later chapter of this book, I give many scriptures people have twisted to satisfy their wicked ways and bad eating habits. I will address many of these commonly misquoted scriptures in that chapter.

However, there is one more issue that needs to be understood concerning animal consumption. We have been given permission to consume animal flesh with restrictions. No matter how many times we ask Yahweh to bless our food, it does not take away those restrictions. Yahweh made our bodies as temples we are to keep clean, free of any toxic things that will harm those vessels.

There are many things that are harmful to our diets which were not around during the time of Yeshua being on earth. Since these things were not known to man at that time, it would have been confusing and irrelevant to mention them. Today, many of these toxic things have become part of our daily lives — for example, the microwave oven. Though the Scriptures never mention microwave ovens, any food prepared in them is harmful towards your health. There are also numerous drugs that are put into foods today that are toxic and should never be in the body. Directly or indirectly, they defile our temples.

Today, countless animals are being overdosed with unnecessary hormones and other toxic drugs. In addition, the food fed to the animals has been grown with toxic chemicals, or the food itself has been mixed with toxic substances. When you consume any animal that has not been raised on a wholesome vegetarian diet, usually grass fed, it is very likely the animal has been fed toxic drugs and even the waste of other animals.

The same is true with many animals being pumped with drugs to fatten them up more quickly and to become bigger than they were meant to be. These toxic drugs are indirectly passed down to us when we consume these animals. If you choose to consume animals, grass fed and organic should be the only way.

Chemical-laden Foods and Soil

Not only animal products, but many of the fruits and vegetables that Yahweh said shall be our food are grown with many toxic chemicals. We hear the word 'organic' often nowadays, but organic foods are nothing new. Organic means chemical free. That's the way Yahweh intended us to eat them. The toxic chemicals added to foods today are very harmful to our health. To make matters worse, much of the produce today is grown in soil that has been sprayed with these chemicals. So just washing the outside of the food won't get rid of many of the toxins that get inside during growth from the toxic soil.

Another major setback is that the soil the food is grown in is no longer rich with minerals that normally would become part of the plant. The decline in the quality of the soil creates low-quality produce. All parts of the process must be high quality for our bodies to get the most out of them. There are so many important nutrients and healing properties within soil.

Most soil today is so depleted of its natural elements that it would be likely the soil Yeshua used to heal the blind man eyes would have very little effect if the quality of the soil were as poor as it is today. I can envision Yeshua being with us today giving us a parable about how we have destroyed the soil, the food, and our health because of our lack of knowledge and lack of desire to comply with His Father's commands.

Hybridized Foods

Do not plant your field with two kinds of seed.
—Leviticus 19:19 [NLT]

The more we transgress from Yahweh's original design, the more we suffer. Because of man's greed, the hybridization of foods today gives us the lowest-quality varieties of crops in our history. It has gotten so out of hand that some people may not even be able to thrive on a vegan diet the way they were originally intended to (Genesis 1:29).

When food is hybridized, the quality of food is lowered, and nutrients are lost. Some plants naturally become hybridized due to natural elements so they can survive. However, man has purposely crossbred plants to grow within each other, mixing the seeds that would never have mixed naturally in nature. This corruption of Yahweh's design produces lower-quality foods and new combinations of old foods making new, much lower-quality varieties in the process.

The big businesses that alter the food for profit claim they do this to make the crop more resistant to diseases due to climate and insect damage. They are just greedy, and the amount of money they can make is more important to them than people's health. They look to see how they can get the most money for the crops, never giving any attention to the quality of food being lost.

Creating new varieties of foods is one example of how the consumer is kept interested and at the same time deceived. Take for example an apricot and a plum. They have been combined, and now we have a pluot. This seems new and exciting, but at what cost to our health?

Another marketing trick is to claim the food is being made easier to eat. For example, because of hybridization, watermelons can no longer produce new seeds within their own food. This adds up to a much lower-quality food, but it is marketed as, wow, watermelon — how much easier to eat with no seeds! And people fall for it.

Watermelon is just an example. There are many fruits that once had lots of seeds that no longer do so. The less work people have to do spitting out the seeds, and the sweeter tasting the food, because we are all addicted to sugar, the more people enjoy this newly created food, but get fewer nutrients out of it.

Most fruits, vegetables, and grains, even when organic, are genetically altered to some degree. The best guideline is to avoid seedless fruits of any kind. People who are unaware of this will not realize that Yahweh has warned us against doing this to the food.

Genetically Modified Foods

Genetically modified (GM) foods are foods that have had their DNA changed through genetic manipulation techniques. Unlike hybrids, which have been created through conventional breeding and have been consumed for thousands of years, genetically modified foods were first put on the market in the early 1990s. The most commonly modified such foods are derived from plants: soybean, corn, canola, and cottonseed oil.

For example, a typical GM food could be a strawberry that has to survive in cold climates. Therefore, the farmer gets its DNA altered so it can survive in the frost. DNA is taken from a frost-resistant cell and transferred into the strawberry cell's genes. Thus the cells of the strawberry are now frost resistant and will survive the frost so that the farmer does not lose money.

This transformation of the food continues the trend of taking us as far as possible, further than we have ever been, from the paradise found in the garden. The crops Yahweh has given as food are no longer the same as He meant them to be. There are long-term health consequences for anyone who is purposely not following Yahweh's guidelines.

People don't realize the potential disaster they are creating once they get in the way of Yahweh's design and try to change it. We contribute to the disaster happening right now by not following His divine schedule, by consuming nonorganic, hybridized, and genetically modified food and supporting the companies that produce them.

Of all the issues with crops today and also with animals, the most common we are seeing more of is the modifying of the seeds and germ cells to produce new, dangerous foods. From corn to fish to tomatoes, scientists are taking the genes of animals and inserting them into the DNA of plant seeds. This has become the world of mad science in the form of what we call food.

Just how bad has it gotten? I have personally cut open a tomato and seen a strawberry grown inside. One day someone will cut open a tomato and find a fish head inside.

The foods currently being genetically modified are soybeans, corn, cotton, Hawaiian papaya, tomatoes, potatoes, sweet corn, rice, rapeseed (canola), sugar cane, sugar beet. It is very important they only be organic if you consume any of these foods. Currently, as of the writing of this book, if these foods are labeled organic, they have not been genetically modified. However, there are more and more battles taking place in the courts to change that and little support to stop the change. So one day, even organic may not safe.

Processed Foods

Of all the foods today, the ones we consume the most often are going to have the biggest impacts on our health. Of the foods Yahweh gave us, the more we get away from the forms in which He gave them to us, the worse our health will be. Foods that are taken out of their original whole states, stripped of their nutrients, fortified with chemicals, and heated to destroy all the enzymes are processed to such a degree they do not even have the same elements that they were meant to.

If you can do anything for your health, cut out the processed foods from your diet. Just about anything that is in a can, bottle, bag, container, box, wrapper is processed to some degree, especially if it has no expiration date on it, and it is sitting on a shelf in a store.

We often see foods mentioned in the Bible, such as bread, that today have been processed to such a degree they are no longer healthful to eat. Some people will claim bread is in the Bible, so it is good for us. I can be sure that Wonder Bread is not the same bread that they were eating in the Bible. Even the grains mentioned in the Bible are no longer the same. Grains such as rice have been stripped of the bran and germ and bleached.

The processed grains are very high on the glycemic index chart, especially when cooked, because they quickly convert to sugar in the bloodstream. This makes most grains and flours poor choices for those in search of health. Wheat products are not a much better choice. Wheat also is usually very processed and contains gluten. Several diseases today are caused by gluten in the diet, including inflammatory bowel disease, also known as ulcerative colitis, Crohn's disease, and celiac disease.

By now I pray you see the point of why so many believers are suffering. Most of their diets consist of processed foods and very little organic produce — all against what Yahweh warned us not to do.

Alcohol Is for the Dying and Wine for Those in Bitter Distress.

Now, therefore, be careful not to drink any wine or other intoxicating liquor, and don't eat anything unclean. —Judges 13:4

If your body is a temple that is to be kept clean and set apart, why would Yahweh want man to defile that temple by putting alcohol into it? The truth is, Yahweh is not against drinking wine for certain occasions, but the amounts and reason it is taken today have created a sinful mess.

I've heard just about every excuse or reason where a so-called believer told me it was okay to drink wine, according to the Scriptures. But the real question here should be why you would even want to. If I had to, I could justify the Scriptures saying it's okay to drink beer. After all, beer is a fermented grain, and the Scriptures support consuming grains. This is foolish reasoning. It's not too much different when people suggest it's okay to drink wine. If you are a believer, truthfully ask yourself why you feel the need to put liquor into your body.

> *Or don't you know that your body is a temple for the Set-apart Spirit who lives inside you, whom you received from Yahweh? The fact is, you don't belong to yourselves;*
>
> *for you were bought at a price. So use your bodies to glorify Yahweh.*
> —1 Corinthians 6:19-20

The real debate that goes on is what wine is according to Yahweh. Is it a fermented drink or a simple, unfermented grape juice? The answer is both. But the result is different. When grape juice is taken, it is healing to the body. When wine is taken, it is bad for health, but also bad for decision making. There is not one place in the Scriptures that fermented wine was taken that resulted in a good situation. You can be sure the wine was unfermented any place in the Scriptures that mentions taking it without a bad result occurring.

Some people may suggest Yeshua's first miracle of making the water into wine was reason to support drinking wine, but this was not about wine being good. It was used as a device for Yeshua to show He was set apart and could give people all they desire.

I don't understand how any believer can think Yeshua could sit there and watch people getting drunk and asking for more wine, and He would say, "Sure, I enjoy this." There is a difference between having one glass of wine with dinner and having extra barrels on hand so the party can last longer. Even one glass may be too much, but no one should ever need more.

> *Stop drinking water; instead, use a little wine for the sake of your digestion and because of your frequent illnesses.* —1 Timothy 5:23

Some people suggest fermented wine is good for the stomach

when they feel unwell. If that's what you believe, take a sip of it as medicine when feeling ill, not as a leisure beverage to put you in a party mood. Fresh-squeezed, unfermented grape juice is always a wiser choice. It is good for the body and will heal a sour stomach much more quickly than liquor. Fermented grape juice or any other fermented sugar will often make the issue worse.

> *Wine is a mocker, strong liquor a rowdy; anyone led astray by it is unwise.* —Proverbs 20:1

Fermentation is a symbol of decay and of sin. How could something that is decaying represent the blood of the spotless Son of Yahweh?

Satan tempts men to indulgence that will cloud reason and numb spiritual perception, but Yeshua teaches us to bring the lower nature into subjection. His whole life was an example of self-denial. It was Yeshua who directed that John the Baptist drink neither wine nor strong drink. There are other warnings in Scripture against drinking wine that will show it is not good or wise.

> *Woe to those who are heroes at drinking wine, men whose power goes to mixing strong drinks.* —Isaiah 5:22

New Wine in Old Bottles

The following text is quoted from the article "The 'I'm Being Religious about Eating' Diet," p. 2-3, Doug Mitchell:

Even among the most sincerely dedicated health reformers, there have been exhibited the results of the age-old proverb

No one puts new wine into old wineskins; if he does, the new wine will burst the skins and be spilled, and the skins too will be ruined. —Luke 5:37

To understand the meaning of this saying, we must look at it in the context of the times in which it was spoken. First, the word translated 'bottles' is actually 'skins', for that was the common item used for storing "new wine." Secondly, the word translated 'wine', when used alone, refers to either fermented or unfermented grape juice. And lastly, the "new wine" was not stored in the skins in order to ferment it into an alcoholic beverage.

Anyone who is familiar with alcoholic winemaking procedures knows that neither bottles nor skins can withstand the gaseous forces given off during the fermenting process. Strong wooden barrels with steel bands are generally used to ferment the grape juice. It is only put into bottles or skins to age after it has fermented because the gases given off during fermentation are gone.

But there was a different use for the skins. They were used to store unfermented grape juice which had first been boiled down to a syrupy consistency. In this state, the grape juice would not ferment when it was sealed and stored in new, unused skins. The problem with putting new wine in a previously used (old) skin was that some of the old grape syrup that was stuck to the insides of the skins would start to ferment when it came into contact with the air. It would thus ferment the new wine it came into contact with, causing the skin to expand until it burst.

Most all of the improvements which people have made in their diets have, unfortunately, been after the manner of the above-quoted adage — that is, they try to bring their new-found principles (the new wine) into their same old incorrect practices (old bottles [skins] with fermented [corrupted] ideas therein). For example, they eat at the customary times, regardless of whether or not those times are the best, and eat in the same manner, regardless of the same.

The science of the cycles of nature, how they affect our digestive processes, and how said processes affect our overall being is an ancient science and must be given its proper place as the foundation of all health. Though we can fairly well train our bodies to accept our choice of eating habits, sooner or later our bad habits will manifest their results in ill health. Long ago a prophet wrote,

Here is what Yahweh says: "Stand at the crossroads and look; ask about the ancient paths, 'Which one is the good way?' Take it, and you will find rest for your souls." —Jeremiah 6:16.

The truths revealed in the "old paths" and "the good way" have become "new wine" to those by whom they are beheld because of their disuse and renewed appreciation. But this situation also has its own obstacle to be overcome.

And no one, having drunk old [wine], *immediately desires new; for he says, "The old is better."* —Luke 5:39 [NKJV]

So the "new wine" — the renewed knowledge of the "old paths" — is at first not desired, because the heart is set upon the path one has been accustomed to.

In examining the customary times of eating, we should consider the source of, and motivation for, their use. Unrealized by most is the fact that religious practices are the basis for the traditional mealtimes. While the original Judeo-Christian times of worship are at the third and ninth hours of the natural day (approximately 9:00 a.m. and 3:00 p.m.), the universal times of worship in ancient sun worship were at the first, sixth, and twelfth hours (approximately 6:00 a.m., 12 noon, and 6:00 p.m.). That meals (feasts) were and are taken in conjunction with times of worship is a well-established fact. Today, the church *potluck* is just one example. It is this physical/spiritual type of meal which has been used to establish the mealtimes, which vary from tradition to tradition.

Commercialism is the other major factor at play in determining mealtimes and the foods which are generally consumed at those times. This is even true of most health food restaurants. Thus, the saying *the love of money is the root of all evil* (1 Timothy 6:10) has application to the improper dietary practices propagated through many commercial food enterprises. There can be no doubt that most restaurants are in business to make money first and secondarily (if at all) to supply people with needed healthful nutrition. There is a high profit margin in the traditional American breakfast foods (eggs, bacon, white bread, pancakes). The same is true of nighttime meals of fancy. And fast food places are generally oriented toward high volumes of low-quality foods for their profits.

There are various ways people attempt to put the *new wine* into *old bottles*. For example, when people decide to replace their customary bacon, eggs, and coffee breakfasts with vegetarian diets (the oldest of "the old paths"), they usually end up eating cereals and fruits for breakfast. Even though health researchers have consistently said that our first meal of the day should be the heartiest, most vegetarians still have their big vegetable meal midday or most commonly in the evening. This is one of the prime reasons why many conscientious folks still suffer from many of the same maladies as those who are indifferent (irreligious) about what, when, and how they eat.

CHAPTER 12

Yahweh's Approved Foods: He Gives Justice to the Oppressed and Food to the Hungry.

So now, Israel, all that Yahweh your Creator asks from you is to fear Yahweh your Creator, follow all His ways, love Him and serve Yahweh your Creator with all your heart and all your being;

to obey, for your own good, the Torah and regulations of Yahweh which I am giving you today. —Deuteronomy 10:12-13

So What's Left to Eat?

Avoiding all the foods that we have become accustomed to enjoying can leave us thinking there is nothing left to eat. We have to understand that Yahweh provides all our needs. He supplies everything we need in abundance. There are a tremendous variety of foods left to consume. The following is a list of the foods that comply with Yahweh's guidelines and are best for our overall health.

Fruits and Vegetables

Then Yahweh said, "Here! Throughout the whole earth I am giving you as food every seed-bearing plant and every tree with seed-bearing fruit." —Genesis 1:29

Some people claim Yahweh changed the original diet of man to include meat. Those who make this claim suggest the intended diet for man was found in the Garden of Eden and consisted of a vegan diet of just fruits and vegetables. Yahweh never changed His plan of what diet man should eat. He gave the first set of instructions, a vegan diet, and later revealed that certain animals are also acceptable as food if someone were to choose it. We cannot overlook that Yahweh always offers His best to us first, and

He first revealed fruit and vegetables as our food. He called it a good thing (Genesis 1:12).

Yahweh intended every nutrient we need to thrive to be found in fruits and vegetables. However, because of the lower-quality produce grown today, it is more challenging in some places to be a vegan without supplementation.

Fruits and vegetables are vital to your health, and everyone needs some in his or her diet to survive. You cannot say that about meat or any other food source. You can leave everything else out of your diet, but fruits and vegetables are a must. Whether you eat an all vegan diet or include some animal products in your diet, we cannot be healthy without eating some amount of produce.

Finding produce ripe, fresh, and organic is important, so we should all do our best to eat all fruits and vegetables this way.

Plant gardens, and eat what they produce. —Jeremiah 29:5

We are more herbivorous (herb-eating) creatures than carnivorous (meat-eating) ones. Our hands are made for picking fruit; our minds are made for planting and growing; our organs are made to digest fruits and herbs. Our teeth are made to chew fruits and vegetables. The gastric juices in our stomachs have to work harder and longer to digest animal food. When it comes to food, fruits and vegetables should be our first choice and the majority of our diets.

Eat Them Raw

Our bodies have been designed to digest fruit and vegetables best when they are uncooked. When food is heated to a temperature above 105°F, many important nutrients, including enzymes, proteins, and many vitamins and minerals, are destroyed. For ultimate health, at least 75% of your diet should consist of raw foods.

When we eat food lacking in enzymes, the body has to expend a tremendous amount of energy digesting the food and then cleansing the body of the waste. When we cook, we're actually taking a high-quality food and making it a lower-quality one.

Cooking also dehydrates the food, taking out the important water and nutritious liquid.

Eat Them Ripe!

When fruit isn't ripe, it hasn't had the chance to develop everything that was intended to be in it for health purposes. There are no fruits that can ripen as properly as it would if it were still on the vine or tree. The unripeness of prematurely picked fruit can be a big issue when trying to eat more healthfully. It is not usually possible to get truly tree ripened fruit, but still make sure you eat fruits when they have fully ripened, even if ripened off the tree. Many fruits that are consumed unripe can be very acidic to the body, creating a toxic internal environment.

Eat Them Fresh!

Getting your food as fresh as possible is also important when it comes to quality. How much time passes since the food was picked from the ground or the tree before you eat it? The distance the food had to be shipped doesn't matter as much as how fresh it is (but that would often make it out of season, another issue). Chances are the food will be fresher if locally grown, but that's not always the case. Find out when it was picked, and do your best to eat foods that are as fresh as possible.

When we cook foods, we lose enzymes. But even when our foods are uncooked, the longer they're sitting somewhere after being picked and before being consumed, the less enzyme activity they'll have. Once picked, all foods start to lose nutrients. Any improvement in the quality of our food will result in an improvement in our health.

Eat them Organic!

I used to think organic meant the peel wasn't sprayed and that if you were to peel or shell the conventionally grown fruit, vegetable, nut, or seed, it would be safe. I've learned that it goes way beyond that. The nonorganic, or conventional, food is grown in soil that is very toxic, which in turn yields toxic produce.

Another big issue with nonorganic foods has to do with the

mineral content of the soil. Vitamins mostly come from the sun and elements above the ground, whereas minerals usually come from the soil and elements beneath the ground. The quality of the food varies widely, depending on the quality of the soil.

This is another reason that even though people say they're vegetarians or raw foodists, they aren't assured of good-quality nutrition. They must make sure to eat high-quality produce. Organically grown is a big factor in this. Once we get some high-quality foods, composting (recycling) the skins and uneaten food will help to assure good-quality soil for future planting.

Live (Rhymes with 'Thrive')

Live foods take raw foods to the next level. They are the highest quality and will do more to benefit our health. Also known as "life foods," they are fermented foods, such as seed cheeses, sauerkraut, yogurt, and other live-cultured foods, along with sprouts, sprouted beans, and grasses. These foods generate predigested proteins and enzymes and maintain the "life force" destroyed by cooking. With live foods, the growing process continues even after the food is picked.

Wild Foods

We cannot buy or even plant the highest-quality foods, but we can get them for free. Common plants and weeds found in people's yards or local parks are mostly edible, and they are the most healthful foods for our bodies. It's important to research which ones are nonedible before exploring wild foods, because they can be poisonous. However, only a small percentage is, while there are hundreds of fascinating, delicious, wild vegetables, fruits, nuts, seeds, and herbs growing in our neighborhoods, backyards, parks, and forests that we overlook and disregard.

Many edible weeds are not too difficult to identify. They are easy to recognize once introduced to them. They are easy to collect and enjoy with no harm to the environment. Many are fine eaten raw, some are better cooked, and many can be dried and stored.

Identifying Wild Plants

Leaves, flowers, fruits, roots, shoots, and thorns all have distinctive characteristics to help assist in identifying edible weeds. Most weeds have flowers attached to them, but they are not very visible to the human eye. A helpful tool in identifying plants would be a magnifying glass.

The color of the little flower heads usually unlocks the mystery of the weed. In identifying leaves, notice that the edges are either sharp or round. Some roots and shoots have small hairs coming out of them, while others are smooth textured.

There are many exciting ways to help identify each weed. Other than a guide or the Internet, the most useful source is a good guidebook. You want to get one that covers the types of weeds that grow in your area, because it is different everywhere. A good guidebook will even say in what region of the country or world the weeds usually grow and where they are usually found, such as near lakes or the seashore, etc.

Some of the more common healthful edible weeds are chickweed, purslane, plantain, lamb's-quarters, and wood sorrel.

Sprouted Food

Unlike wild, edible weeds that take no work by man to grow, sprouted food takes some work, but the food is so nutritious it is well worth it. Sprouted food is any type of seed, nut, grain, or bean that has been soaked in water, exposed to air and indirect sunlight, and when rinsed daily, has started to form a new plant, beginning with a sprout. Some examples include wheatgrass, sunflower sprouts, sprouted almonds, and even bean sprouts. Sprouts are 10 to 30 times more nutritious than the best vegetables, either as is or juiced. They are the most nutritious of all land-based foods.

Vegetables and Salad Greens

Most foods in our diets should come from fresh, chlorophyll-rich, leafy greens. You'll find many in your market or natural food store you may never have heard of before. Try the new ones as often as possible. Here are the more common ones: arugula, bok choy, chicory, collard greens, dandelion, garlic greens, kale, many varieties of lettuce, mustard greens, spinach, Swiss chard, turnip greens, watercress, sunflower greens.

Other vegetables that should be a good part of our diet are asparagus, broccoli, cabbage, cauliflower, celery, green (string) beans.

Chlorophyll-rich green, leafy vegetables are blood builders. According to the Scriptures, "The life of a creature is in the blood," as stated in Leviticus 17:11. Leviticus 17:11 is more in reference to our spiritual health. The blood of Yeshua will save us spiritually, but since the quality of our blood also will determine whether we are healthy or sick, the same scripture can be used in reference to our physical health.

Nobel Peace Prize winner Dr. Otto Warburg confirms this. The quality of our blood will determine the quality of our health. The quality of your blood is the foundation for a healthy body.

> Blood sustains the entire body organ in nutrient delivery and waste management. Blood streams through the vascular system, throughout the arteries, away from the heart to arterioles to capillaries and returns via veins to the heart once again. As long as the body has adequate oxygen and the body fluid and tissue have an acid/alkaline balance, amazing health ensues. —*Secrets of an Alkaline Body* by David and Annie Jubb.

There is much talk today about pH levels, alkaline/acid percentages, etc. When it comes to clean blood and dirty blood, it gets quite confusing. To me, the best way to describe it is that dirty blood will cause poor health because it lacks sufficient oxygen. Clean blood is blood that has a sufficient amount of oxygen.

Most poor-quality foods today, eaten in poor-quality forms, will clog the bloodstream with much waste, leading to a lack of oxygen in the bloodstream. Blood carries nutrients to all parts of the body; it also carries oxygen to all parts of the body.

A lack of oxygen in the bloodstream creates the environment

for fungus to grow: candida, as well as cancer cells. These cells can thrive only in a poorly oxygenated environment. Clean, well-oxygenated blood will clean up the problem. Poor health is the result of dirty blood. In my opinion, every illness — from candida to cancer and everything in between — is caused by oxygen-deficient, dirty blood. If the blood is toxic, it won't be able to do its job efficiently, and this is where the problems continue to worsen. Because most people today are eating against the way Yahweh told us, most people have this loss of oxygen in their bloodstreams.

Yahweh didn't make errors in creating our bodies wonderful and amazing. He gave us all we need to keep our blood clean. But as we stray away from His Torah, we fill our bodies with slime, mucus, and toxins that go against Yahweh's plan for us. Ultimately, we dirty our blood, causing all sorts of later stages of disease.

How do we reverse the problem and get the oxygen into the body? Yahweh gives us the answer. Most people today eat too much processed, low-quality food, full of fat and sugar. They also consume too much protein. Eating this way is not part of Yahweh's instructions.

His dietary instructions say the majority of our diets should be chlorophyll-rich green vegetables, herbs, algae, sea vegetables, and sprouts. All these foods are excellent according to Yahweh's Torah, but people eat too little of these foods. If we want to experience the blessings of Yahweh's Torah, we need to make sure the majority of our diets consist of these foods.

The reason these green foods are so beneficial for the body is that they contain chlorophyll. Chlorophyll is the green pigment of the plants. It is also known as the blood of plants. It is almost identical to hemoglobin, the pigment that colors our blood red and carries oxygen into our cells. Chlorophyll has been used in blood transfusion successfully at times of emergency.

In taking chlorophyll into the body, vital oxygen is also taken in. This is why wheatgrass is used at so many health spas around the world in the treatment of cancer and other deadly diseases. The greener the leaf, the more chlorophyll it has. Sea algae are available in several edible forms that contain a great deal of chlorophyll as well. Green foods also contain a large amount of minerals lacking in other foods.

Yahweh told us to use the foods that are best for us and that green, leafy herbs are our medicine.

I find it interesting that of all the times Yahweh mentions food in the Bible, the only time He said it was good was in Genesis 1:12.

> *The earth brought forth grass, plants each yielding its own kind of seed, and trees each producing its own kind of seed-bearing fruit; and Yahweh saw that it was good.* —Genesis 1:12

All other times, He says what's allowed in our diet, but doesn't say what's good. So if we are eating a diet consisting of mostly green, leafy vegetables, we can take care of our nutritional needs, and Yahweh said it is good. An important reminder is that no matter what food we eat, if we are overdoing it, or making an idol out of it, the result can turn negative for our health.

Fruits

Any plant containing a seed is technically a fruit. The more liquid a fruit has, the better it is for you usually, because the easier it is to digest. Melons have the most liquid of all fruits and digest most easily. There are many fruits that are commonly considered to be vegetables, but since they contain a seed, they are a fruit. This would include tomatoes, cucumbers, zucchini, and bell peppers. Of all the foods for man, fruit is the most natural and digests the most easily.

Nuts and Seeds

Nuts and seeds are best eaten after they have been soaked for 6 to 12 hours because soaking releases enzymes that allow for easier digestion. It's very easy to eat too many nuts, so be careful. However, nuts and seeds both provide a great variety and source of nutrients, so include them in your diet.

Sea Vegetables

Sea vegetables are very high in both the major minerals and trace minerals (which help the electrical frequencies of the body and the immunity of the body, etc.). Sea vegetables are the most nutritious foods in the ocean. There are many different types of sea vegetables.

When I was a kid walking on the beach on Coney Island in Brooklyn, New York, I saw something that I never thought would become one of my main nutrient sources years later. As the waves would come ashore and subside, they would often leave clumps of seaweeds on the wet sand. Forget about eating it! I didn't even want to step in it.

It wasn't until many years later that I found myself at Hippocrates Health Institute in West Palm Beach, Florida, stricken with a deadly disease. I found myself learning about a new way of eating: the raw vegan diet. And a big part of the HHI diet was — you guessed it — seaweeds.

It took me awhile to get used to eating the many different types of seaweeds, but as I learned how good and healthful they were for me, it became a lot easier. Many raw food recipes included seaweeds, which even made the dishes taste a lot better.

Over the years, I have come to depend on them for my minerals and nutrients that are no longer found in modern soil that grows fruits and vegetables. There is an abundance of minerals and trace elements in ocean water and on the ocean floor that makes the many varieties of sea vegetables so valuable to us today. I suggest anyone wanting to eat a raw vegan diet to eat a wide variety of sea vegetables. Sea vegetables are one of the richest food sources of minerals and trace elements.

Many sea vegetables also come in powdered, green super foods or capsules to help if you don't have time to eat the actual weeds, or if you don't enjoy the flavor. I assure you that once you make some delicious recipes with seaweeds, the flavor will no longer be an issue.

You may ask yourself why any human would need to consume sea vegetables. It may seem very unnatural to do so. But many of the people who ask this question eat fish, which is even more unnatural. We are living in such a polluted world, and the minerals have been stripped from our soils. Even produce grown in organic soil is not as good as it used to be and should be. By adding sea vegetables to our diets, we are making sure we get the best of the best.

Here are a few of the most popular with their most important benefits:

Alaria

Delicious raw in salads, either presoaked or marinated. Comparable to whole sesame seeds in calcium content (1100mg/100g). Very high vitamin A, comparable to parsley, spinach, or turnip greens; very high in B vitamins.

Arame

Nutty sea vegetable taste. Very high in calcium, phosphorous, iodine, iron, potassium, and vitamins A and B.

Dulse

Delicious as a raw snack, with a distinctive, strong sea flavor. Great in salads. Protein, 22%: more than chickpeas, almonds, or whole sesame seeds. A handful gives a whole day's supply of iron. The same handful will provide more than 100% of the RDA for vitamin B_6. Relatively low in sodium (1740mg/100g), high in potassium (7820mg/100g).

Hijiki

Very high in calcium; vitamins A, B_1, and B_2; and phosphorous.

Kelp

Tastes great marinated. Exceptionally high in all major minerals, particularly calcium, potassium, magnesium, and iron. Rich in important trace minerals, such as manganese, copper, and zinc. One ounce of kelp provides the recommended daily dose of chromium, instrumental in blood sugar regulation. That same ounce provides many times the RDA for iodine, essential to the thyroid gland and lacking in many terrestrial soils.

Nori

Distinctive mild, nutty, salty-sweet taste. Great in salads and can be used to make vegetable nori rolls. Protein, 28%: more than sunflower seeds, lentils, or wheat germ. An excellent source of naturally occurring manganese, fluoride, copper, and zinc. Of all the sea vegetables, nori is the highest in vitamins B_1, B_2, B_6, C, and E.

Whole Grains and Legumes

It's best to eat grains that have been sprouted first, so they are easier to digest. The least healthful grains are rye, spelt, basmati rice, white rice, wheat, barley, and corn. The most healthful grains are millet, quinoa, amaranth, teff, buckwheat (hulled).

Milk, Cheese, Eggs, and Honey

> *He swore to your ancestors to give you a land flowing with milk and honey.* —Exodus 13:5

The Scriptures talk about all of these foods in a positive way, but do not give direct instructions about them. Raw milk from goats or sheep is excellent for health. However, milk purchased today from the supermarket is usually processed, cooked (pasteurized), homogenized, and loaded with chemicals. If that is the only milk you can get, avoid it. Also, milk from a cow is not ideal because a baby calf grows to be 800 pounds, and the cow will produce a composition of the milk to support such a large animal. This milk has too much protein and fat for humans to consume and is very mucus forming.

However, a baby goat or sheep grows to be about the same size as a human, and the milk very closely resembles a human mother's milk. Getting the milk raw is not easy because many laws ban the sale of raw animal milk. Also, too much of the milk can be a little mucus forming. The milk is not needed, but it can be helpful if you cannot get a full range of nutrients from other sources because of income or location. If you choose to consume milk, make sure it is raw goat or sheep milk only. Milk from grass-fed animals is best.

Honey

Honey is mentioned several times in the Scriptures and was a very special treat for some, but a main source of food for others, such as John the Baptist. Honey today is just as nutritious, but because of the high amount of sugar in most people's diets, the added sugar from honey can be too much. Only consume honey if you do not eat a lot of other sugar in your diet. All honey should be consumed raw.

Eggs

Eggs are good.

> *Or if he asked for an egg, would give him a scorpion?* —Luke 11:12

Eggs are an excellent food that Yeshua suggests in the above scripture are good things. If you do choose to consume eggs, make sure they come from organic, free range, nonanimal-fed chickens.

Overall, the most healthful way to consume an egg is raw. If the taste of a raw egg is not so desirable, adding it to a milkshake or smoothie gives you all the benefits without the taste.

Clean Meats

> *These are the living creatures which you may eat among all the land animals:*
>
> *any that has a separate hoof which is completely divided and chews the cud — these animals you may eat.* —Leviticus 11:2-3

We have already read that if any meat or other animal product is consumed, it should be free range, organic, and considered clean by Yahweh. The blood and the fat should never be consumed. Because animal flesh is very hard to digest, we should limit the amount of meat consumed.

During the times the Scriptures were written, the average Torah follower, unless he had a lot of money, ate meat only during the high holy days and special appointed feast days and celebrations, about three or four times a year. History shows these people lived longer than people who could afford to consume meat much more often. If you choose to consume meat, it would be wise to limit it to no more than three or four times a month and in small amounts. The more often you are going to consume it, the less you should eat within each meal.

If you do enjoy eating animal flesh, here are the animals that are clean to eat according to Yahweh: cow, deer, lamb, buffalo, elk, goat, moose, and caribou.

Fish

Of all the things that live in the water, you may eat these: anything in the water that has fins and scales, whether in seas or in rivers — these you may eat. —Leviticus 11:9

Fish was a common food all throughout the biblical times. If it is gotten from clean water, it is still an excellent food today. We need to be careful not to eat it too much or too often. Some clean fish according to the Torah are bass, bluefish, crappie, perch, pike, salmon, sunfish, trout. However, keep in mind that just because it's clean according to the Torah, that doesn't make it immune to the toxins in the ocean that would make the fish unhealthful to consume.

Birds

You may eat any bird that is ceremonially clean.
—Deuteronomy 14:11 [NLT]

Birds would fall into the same category as meat. Here are the birds that are ceremonially clean: chicken, turkey, grouse, quail.

Clean Creeping Animals

Specifically, of these you may eat the various kinds of locusts, grasshoppers, katydids, and crickets. —Leviticus 11:22

Most people in the United States never consume insects intentionally, but it is common in other parts of the world. The most common approved insects that are okay to eat according to the Scriptures are locusts, crickets, and grasshoppers.

CHAPTER 13

Beyond Diet: Supplements and Herbs. Life Is More than Just Bread Alone

Supplements

When we eat according to the Scriptures, it may seem that we can get all the required nutrients from our diet. However, with poor-quality soil and preconditioned sicknesses already existing amongst us in today's world, there are times when taking supplements in addition to our food can be vital to our health.

We have to do our best to find food that is as high in quality as possible. If it's not available, I suggest taking high-quality supplements to make up for any possible deficiency. I don't feel that eating low-quality foods that Yahweh warned us not to eat is the answer.

But what supplements we need and how much we need should not be decided upon based on what we feel we need. Everyone should have his blood checked at least once a year and let the blood profile reveal what nutrients are lacking. If a person is eating a correct diet in the right amounts and at the ideal times and is still deficient in any nutrient, it is time for supplementation.

Too many people today run to the store blindly taking vitamins and herbs without knowing much about them or whether they are even needed. This can result in a waste of money and can even lead to toxicity if they are not needed but taken. I never suggest vitamins to anyone until I view the blood profile first to see what nutrients exactly are missing. I would also suggest a person get nutrients from food first. If that does not help the issue, taking a good quality supplement usually can resolve it.

Herbs are great medicine to our body, but we should take herbs only to treat or prevent an issue. Herbs should never be taken "because they said it was good." What's good for one person is not always good or even necessary for the next.

Supplements for Disease

Each disease requires a different program. For people who are already dealing with later stages of disease, certain supplements can save their lives. Many people who are sick are very malnourished and need massive amounts of nutrients. A person cannot always got the required nutrients from food soon enough. Also supplements taken orally may not be enough. There are other methods for getting the nutrients into the system more quickly, such as intravenously through a drip line. Sometimes known as liquid vitamins, this should only be performed under supervision and if needed.

CHAPTER 14

Misunderstood Scriptures about Food and Diet: The Wise Shall Understand

For it doesn't go into his heart, but into his stomach, and it passes out into the latrine. —Mark 7:19

Thus he declared all foods ritually clean.

Of all the scriptures about food, no scripture is as misunderstood as Mark 7:19. The confusion is because this text is mistranslated. Most modern versions added, "In saying this, Yeshua declared all foods clean." However, this added sentence was never in early translations of Scripture. Yeshua never declared all foods okay to eat. Yeshua taught every day out of the Torah. He commanded everyone to obey the instructions in Torah and all things including diet. This verse wasn't even a reference about diet. Food here was used as a metaphor. This is clearly an attempt by gentile or Christian editors to abandon Torah's dietary rules.

The real point of that scripture is that if you plot things like murder, lying, adultery, and so forth, then why be concerned about the food you eat when weightier things are making you much more unclean than your food? Even if a person kept a perfectly clean diet but had such unclean thoughts, such a one would rank among the most unclean of people.

The real lesson of this scripture verse was the issue of the whole chapter of Mark 7. Yeshua was teaching about how the Pharisees and scribes have all these man-made laws about how to live and used their man-made laws about diet as an example.

The lesson had nothing to do with food. Yeshua was stating His disagreement with the Pharisees and scribes about how they were so careful to follow the traditions of man but had no concern for the instructions of Yahweh. Thus He was stating your heart must be touched for you to change your evil ways, and food, clean or unclean, means nothing if your heart stays the same.

We are told in Scripture not to change any verse or add or subtract the meaning. By adding to the verse that Yeshua declared all foods acceptable to eat and thereby confusing many, the translators are clearly the ones who are committing an abomination to Yahweh's Word.

> *Every moving thing that lives will be food for you; just as I gave you green plants before, so now I give you everything.* —Genesis 9:3

Many people claim this scripture says it's okay to eat all animals, but they do not read the next verse that says, "But you must never eat any meat that still has the lifeblood in it." They also do not take into account Leviticus and Deuteronomy, which state the full restrictions that come with eating animals.

> *I looked inside and saw four-footed animals, beasts of prey, crawling creatures and wild birds.*
> *Then I heard a voice telling me, "Get up, Peter, slaughter and eat!"*
> *I said, "No, sir! Absolutely not! Nothing unclean, or tref, has ever entered my mouth!"*
> *But the voice spoke again from heaven: "Stop treating as unclean what Yahweh has made clean."* —Acts 11:6-9

All believers, Jewish or not, are called never to eat unclean things according to Leviticus 11 and Deuteronomy 14. This scripture does not change that. This scripture was not about that issue. The real meaning is about gentile converts who were turning to Yahweh. New converts were not to be viewed as unclean.

> *Well, whatever you do, whether it's eating or drinking or anything else, do it all so as to bring glory to Yahweh.* —1 Corinthians 10:31

Some mistake this scripture, thinking they can consume any food they want as long as they praise Yahweh before eating. You cannot please Yahweh by eating things that He has ordained unclean and unholy.

> *The Spirit clearly says that in later times some will abandon the faith and follow deceiving spirits and things taught by demons.*
>
> *Such teachings come through hypocritical liars, whose consciences have been seared as with a hot iron.*
>
> *They forbid people to marry and order them to abstain from certain foods which Yahweh created to be received with thanksgiving by those who believe and who know the truth.*
>
> *For everything Yahweh created is good, and nothing is to be rejected if it is received with thanksgiving,*
>
> *because it is consecrated by the word of Yahweh and prayer.*
> —1 Timothy 4:1-5 [NIV]

Everything Yahweh created is good for a reason, but not everything is good for eating! Many people take this scripture out of context. Everything it says it true, but making it fit our theories does not make our theories correct.

Yahweh clearly tells us what foods are clean and what foods are unclean. The unclean foods are strictly forbidden! No prayer will change that. Saying a prayer over unclean food doesn't sanctify the food any more than praying that you don't get caught stealing can "sanctify" or protect you from the consequences of that transgression. Just because punishment is not always immediate doesn't mean that it's been forgotten.

The Choice is up to you!

I call on heaven and earth to witness against you today that I have presented you with life and death, the blessing and the curse. Therefore, choose life, so that you will live, you and your descendants. —Deuteronomy 30:19

The apostle Paul tells us that no matter how many choices we have and no matter how appealing they may seem to our human eyes and understanding, we should never settle for any choice other than which is Yahweh's will for us.

I told you earlier in this book that you could replace the word 'evil' in the Scriptures many times with the word 'sickness', and it would be a perfect fit. The word 'proverb' means 'wisdom'. This is a book about health according to the Scriptures. Yahweh tells us over and over again in the Scriptures through examples, testimonials, and history that as long as people have faith in Him and fear Him, they will be blessed. There is no greater wisdom in the world. If you want to be healthy, fear Yahweh!

The fear of Yahweh leads to life; one who has it is satisfied and rests untouched by evil. —Proverbs 19:23

And the Scriptures are Yahweh's treasure map to lead us to that treasure!

Yahweh gave us guidelines and instructions (Torah) because He loves us, and we do our best to obey His instructions because we love Him. In fact, "This is the love of Yahweh, that we keep His commandments" (1 John 5:3). Therefore, obeying even the least of the instructions in the Torah is clearly following the teachings of Yeshua.

No matter how long it takes and no matter how many times you stumble, stay focused and faithful, and Yahweh will direct your path. This is a book about health vs. disease. The path that Yahweh wants us on is the path of health. An obedient heart is the path to health. Have faith in Yahweh, and He will show you a more excellent way!

PART 3

Divine Design — Yahweh's Schedule

CHAPTER 15

How We Were Designed to Eat: Do Not Add to or Take Away from His Words on How to Eat

The righteous person eats his fill, but the belly of the wicked is empty.
—Proverbs 13:25

Believers should eat to live, not live to eat. Becoming aware of the things we discussed already, ideal eating times and correct foods may have been something you heard about at some point in the past but just didn't put into practice. However, there is a more basic lesson found in the Scriptures about our eating patterns that very few people ever give thought to. This is because it is such a basic element of life: how we eat.

In addition to instructions about what and when we should eat, the Scriptures instruct us how to eat. This may seem childish because when we were babies, we were taught this basic natural lesson. We all know how to eat, but most of us eat the wrong way. Chances are that our parents didn't eat according to the guidelines found in the Scriptures, and we learned their bad habits. These are more ways man has gotten away from the instructions of Yahweh. They are just as important as everything else we have discussed thus far.

- Don't overeat
- Chew your food well
- Follow food combining
- Eat in a good environment
- Observe a Sabbath year for land

Overeating

We should not eat until we are full.

> *He lets his face grow gross and fat, and the rest of him bulges with blubber.* —Job 15:27

The Scriptures tell us not only what kinds of food we should eat, but also how much food we should eat. Additionally, how often we should eat is a very important topic that many people overlook because of lack of knowledge, deception, or addiction. Regardless of the reason, most people today eat too much and too often.

What is too much food? Technically, consuming more food than our bodies have a nutritional need for is too much. So we shouldn't consume more than our nutritional needs.

When we consume the high-quality foods outlined in the Torah, we will meet our nutritional needs and feel satisfied emotionally. However, if we eat lower-quality food or unscriptural foods, or if we eat for inappropriate reasons (such as emotional comfort), we will overeat. When we eat more than we need, then instead of efficiently doing its work of digestion, the body has to work harder and spend extra time trying to eliminate the extra waste. This overeating, along with eating foods that are not healthful for us, can become a very dangerous mix.

> *Do not carouse with drunkards or feast with gluttons, for they are on their way to poverty.* —Proverbs 23:20-21 [NLT]

It amazes me that members of assemblies (churches) are often quick to identify a person who drinks too much alcohol and hastily condemn him, but a glutton goes largely unnoticed. You don't just have to attend a church barbecue or spend a lot of time with someone out of the church to see a member overindulge himself in all sorts of meals. Often after a church service when food is served, you can view more people interested in the food than they were in the message. The person usually indulging the most is the pastor or other church leader.

To make matters worse, the food or drink usually being served is coffee and donuts or some other unhealthful food, certainly not food found in the Garden of Eden. It bewilders me how many churches today have their own coffee shops as part of the church. They charge people for food most of the time, but often it's an all-you-can-eat-for-free contest after service. The bigger the church, the bigger the budget and the more food usually offered.

People have always overeaten, but because of a lack of exercise (another harmful result of laziness), the results of harmful eating and gluttony are beginning to show much sooner. Eating a diet that goes against Scripture isn't a new fad. Proper diet has been ignored for a long time, and disease has continued to rise.

The reason people suffer more from overeating today than they did before is because the quality of the food is getting worse, because people have more money to overindulge, and because of modern discoveries that we call conveniences, all of which contribute to our laziness.

During the times of scriptural history, it was much more difficult to become overweight. You had to walk many places or ride a horse. Not many people had money to obtain excess food, and there weren't so many modern machines that make it easy for people to be overweight.

The stomach is supposed to be the size of your fist, and your fist is not supposed to be big and fat. The layers of fat on top of your belly are not your stomach. They are layers of fat on your stomach area. Think about how much work the body has to do when we eat large meals and eat very often. We have taken a simple daily blessing from Yahweh (nourishment) and turned it into a daily sin (gluttony).

King Solomon had wisdom about having more than we need:

> *Keep falsehood and futility far from me, and give me neither poverty nor wealth. Yes, provide just the food I need today;*
>
> *for if I have too much, I might deny You and say, "Who is Yahweh?" And if I am poor, I might steal and thus profane the name of my Creator.* —Proverbs 30:8-9

These verses show King Solomon asking for neither too much nor too little of anything, just enough according to Yahweh's will. This request includes regarding food. King Solomon understood that too little of the necessities of life can be harmful, and too much can be just as bad. So he prayed for just enough.

We can see other examples in the Scriptures of how the sin of overeating led to man's destruction.

> *The crimes of your sister Sodom were pride and gluttony; she and her daughters were careless and complacent, so that they did nothing to help the poor and needy.*
>
> *They were arrogant and committed disgusting acts before Me; so that when I saw it, I swept them away.* —Ezekiel 16:49-50

In those verses, Yahweh tells about them being haughty and committing pride, speaks of their fullness of bread, and relates that there was an abundance of idleness.

Fullness of bread is listed as being one of the sins of Sodom, and it is listed near the beginning of the list. "Fullness of bread" can also be translated as "fullness from food." When we eat until we are so full, we create sickness and disease in our bodies. We are not to eat until we are full; rather, we should stop short of fullness.

More scriptures talk about the sin of overeating and man's selfish ways.

> *When he has filled his belly, Yahweh will vent His burning anger against him and rain down His blows upon him.* —Job 20:23 [NIV]
>
> *Because his appetite would not let him rest, in his greed, he let nothing escape.* —Job 20:20
>
> *In the midst of plenty, he will run into trouble, and disasters will destroy him.* —Job 20:22 [NLT]

These verses talk about the connection between filling our bellies (overeating) and the distress that comes along with it. Eating against Yahweh's guide will not only bring disease and sickness to our lives, but will also shorten our lives.

> *Let your moderation be known unto all men. Yahweh is at hand.*
> —Philippians 4:5 [KJV]

There are a goodly number of scriptures that direct us to practice moderation in all good things, and this includes food and drink. (We should completely avoid things that are not good.) Overeating causes stress that causes the body to work harder. When you create more of a workload for your body than it can handle, the result is stress. Too much of any food or drink, good or bad, will create stress in the body leading to poor health.

Overeating creates havoc in the body, causing improper digestion and improper elimination. When the large intestine retains food longer than it should, harmful bacterial action occurs. The result is that gases and toxins are formed. They are absorbed by the tiny vessels on the walls of the bowel and poison the entire bloodstream. This is known as autointoxication.

If you are a big eater, put a knife to your throat. —Proverbs 23:2

Can our bodies run out of room for the extra food? Where does it go? There is a reason why the most developed countries around the world have the most obese people living there. All the extra food that is consumed becomes fat on the body.

The extra fat can turn into a deadly weapon if it gets too out of control. It usually does. Heart disease is the number one cause of death in most developed countries around the world. And other causes of death, such as cancer, diabetes, and strokes have direct connections with too much eating.

Look at it this way: If you have an empty room and keep filling it up with stuff, there will no longer be room for any more stuff once the space runs out. If you keep trying to put more stuff into it, ignoring the fact that there just isn't any more room, eventually the stuff in the room will overflow and come out any way it can — through windows, doors, or any opening it can find. If the openings are blocked, the walls might even break and crumble.

The body works a similar way. The more you eat, the more room you take up in your body. The bad food you eat clogs the body's openings, and this excess waste has nowhere to go. That's when the body will start to crumble, just like the walls of the room.

No matter how good or bad the food you eat, it will be harmful to the body if you eat too much. It will cause your body to work harder than it can, leading to loss of energy. That will lead to many other health problems.

Your body uses what it needs and attempts to dispose of what it doesn't require. Consuming low-quality food makes it more challenging for your body to do the job it was designed to do. We have already discussed the foods that shouldn't be consumed if we are going to listen to Yahweh's direction. There are some people who overindulge even when eating the correct foods, but the majority of people who overeat are those who eat the taboo foods. This is because those foods do not have the nutrients the body requires, so even though the person eating them is still not getting the required nutrients, that person will crave more food.

Most people in the United States overeat. If no one in this country overate, the phrase "I don't like that" wouldn't be in the English language. Anything and everything would taste wonderful to you — if you were really eating with true hunger. People in this country and throughout much of the world don't eat out of hunger; they eat for pleasure. Don't focus on not overeating; there is nothing wrong with a little pleasure. A little pleasure has never hurt anyone. However, a lot of pleasure has killed many.

Learn to control your pleasure. You must gain control. It's fine to experience the pleasure of food, but overdoing it turns into overeating. Learn to ensure that all your nutrient needs are met while reducing your food intake to the amount needed. The right amount of food is different for everyone, but you can be sure that the higher the quality of the food (the closer it is to nature), the less food will be needed.

When you become a believer, you should hate the things of the past that controlled you and led you into sin. You should hate your old lifestyle, and every fiber of your being should joyfully seek to please Yahweh and fulfill His requests. As perfect as this plan seems, our hearts may be willing, but our flesh can be weak. We have been living with the habit of overeating all our lives, and to stop overnight seems impossible. However, nothing is impossible with Yahweh. We can do all things with Him who strengthens us. The best way to break the addictive habit of overeating is to pray. While praying, repent for yielding to the temptation of lust, or food and drink, and ask Yahweh to help you overcome the addiction.

Giving up the action is only half the battle. Your body may go through some sort of natural cleanse, and you may not feel your best during this time. Do not worry. When you eat less than you usually do, you might get a headache or feel weak. This is not caused by a lack of food, but rather by old toxins being loosened into your bloodstream. Eating, because it requires the expenditure of energy for digestion, stops your body from cleansing, and thus stops the old toxins from being released.

It might feel good to stop discomfort this way, but it's very harmful over time because all the toxins continue to build up in the body. When you eat something, it might seem that the food is energizing, but this can be due to the food's stimulating properties and not to the food's strengthening power. Overeating forces your body to use much energy; it does not give your body greater amounts of energy, despite the stimulating effect.

The way to conserve healing energy and build strength is either to eat very little or to fast, depending on your level of health. This will give your system a chance to clean itself, to dislodge and get rid of poisons stored in the body, to get rid of disease, and to heal.

It's not the amount of food that keeps you alive; it's the amount of food your body can use. Any excess will just cause trouble. You can eat a lot of food and still starve to death if your cells cannot use anything in the food. It's not how much you eat, but how much of what you eat the body can use.

The amount of nutrients each person needs will vary on an individual basis. Most people overconsume, and more is not necessarily better because it produces waste. It is this waste that causes many diseases today. There are of course spiritual causes of disease, but from an eating standpoint, disease is either the result of a deficiency or detoxification. Many people think they're getting too little when in fact they're getting too much.

Two other important factors are how toxic a person is and the quality of the foods eaten. The more toxic people are, the more they might feel the continuous need to eat. If they go without food, they'll feel very sick. This is usually not a sign that they need more nutrition, but a good sign that they need less. The reason they feel so sick is that the body is trying to clean out. Once they eat, they usually *feel* better, but they are just stopping the body's natural cleansing process. The fact is, the cleaner people are internally and the higher the quality of their food intake, the less they will need to consume, and their bodies will get much more out of it.

We can enjoy eating the correct foods. They were made for us. But we should not abuse this freedom and hurt ourselves. Drinking too much leads to alcoholism; gluttony leads to obesity. Be careful that what our Creator has provided for your enjoyment doesn't grow into a bad habit that takes control over you.

> *If you obey, you will enjoy a long life in the land.*
> —Deuteronomy 11:9 [NLT]

Yahweh instructs us to avoid bad company. A saved person should not enjoy the company of unbelievers. When we are in the company of the unsaved, there is more of a temptation for us to slip back to our old, addictive habits. This is why we are told in Proverbs not eat with gluttons.

Chew Your Food Well

We have gotten so far away from Yahweh's eating plan that many of us have even forgotten why we have been created the way we have. Each body part was created for a reason, and we have teeth to chew our food! People seem to forget this important step when eating. Digestion begins in the mouth, and if we grind our food into a liquid before we swallow it, we create even less work for our digestive system, making it easier for the body to extract the nutrients from the food.

Chewing, or *mastication*, stimulates the salivary glands to release saliva, which begins to act on the food immediately, breaking it down before it even makes its way to the stomach. Chew your food thoroughly into a creamy consistency. In addition, eating large amounts of food without chewing sufficiently means real difficulty for the intestines to digest and then assimilate the nutrients from the food. We need to make sure all food is in liquid form before swallowing it.

Some foods require more chewing than others, such as more dense foods, so I am not going to suggest the number times one should chew each bite, but a good rule to keep in mind would be to chew your drinks and drink your foods. This is the best way to assure mixing your food very well with salvia before it is swallowed. Don't talk with food in your mouth.

If you're tired of all that chewing, or you just need a break from it, or you just happen to like smoothies, blended soups, and juices, there are other ways to eat that don't require so much chewing: juicing and blending. Both methods can save your body some energy, but still remember you must mix the liquid with saliva in your month well before swallowing. So swirl it around in your month and enjoy the flavors before gulping it down.

Food Combining

Yahweh designed each food to grow in a certain area. If we ate only the foods in a certain area, we would naturally be eating food that digests well with other foods. These combinations of foods, which Yahweh designed to be consumed in a way that will permit the body to enjoy the easiest possible digestion, will help conserve our vital energy.

However, a common issue today is that we have the capability to get foods from all over the world and eat them at the same time. Too many different types of foods in one meal can create poor food combining, something Yahweh's design never intended.

Mixing the wrong foods together or eating them in the wrong order can zap energy and cause fermentation and putrefaction. Proper food combining is a way to eat that allows for easier digestion and minimal digestive conflicts.

It works like this: Every food takes a certain amount of time to digest. Eating similar foods with similar digestive times helps the body digest meals more easily. These foods are said to combine well. For example, watermelon takes about one hour to digest; almonds may take up to five hours. In view of this, eating watermelon and almonds at the same meal is not a good idea. It's known as a poor combination. Eating too many meals like this will cause constipation, bloating, and gas, which could lead to more serious issues.

Since there are different types of raw foods, each with its unique digestive time, your body will have to work harder to digest foods eaten in poor combinations. Ideally, you'd want your body to use as little power as possible for digestion — the very reason it's important to combine your foods properly.

There are people who can mix their foods and not have problems, but many can't; so I recommend heeding correct food combining rules, and if possible, sequential eating. I suggest placing the food combining chart on page 129 on your refrigerator door.

Eat in a Good Environment

A large number of the Jewish people did not use chairs when eating. They lay down on the floor when they ate as a sign of freedom and also as a symbol of a stress-free environment. We see this example during the last supper. I am not suggesting we need to sit on the floor when we eat, but the idea is that when we are stressed in any manner, eating is not healthy. It's okay to skip a meal if you must, but of all the bad eating habits people have today, eating while stressed is one of the most harmful and also one of the most common.

Understanding Nutritional Categories

Health doesn't begin with what we add to the diet; it's what we leave out that's important! That's why many of the popular trendy diets today seem to be okay and get results, because this is what they all have in common: they all leave out something harmful. Only when you find a diet that leaves out not just some, but all, of the harmful foods, will you experience health in the long run, not just for short-term results.

Your physical health mirrors your diet. Your spiritual health mirrors your dis-ease, or your disobedience. Eating higher-quality foods will give you higher-quality health. Eating lower-quality foods will give you lower-quality health. Whatever you decide to eat, obedience to Yahweh is most important. Today's public disregard of health and nutrition is alarming, but more alarming is the rejection of Yahweh's Word. Most popular diets are opposite from the diet Yahweh guided us to eat in His Scriptures.

Commonly today, people think the nutritional categories are fats, sugars, proteins, and carbohydrates. The advertisers deceive the public into buying whatever source of food they will make the most money from, and people are falling for it.

Many people are making the same mistake that Joshua made, as we discussed earlier in this book: they don't consult Yahweh to discern if a product is good for them or not. Instead, they rush out to get the next trendy food spoken about in a health magazine or television commercial. Yahweh didn't make foods with labels on them, and it is not natural to have to read labels and use that as our way to discern if a food is healthful or not. We should be reading our Scriptures instead. That will give us the true answer.

Observing a Sabbath Rest of the Land

When you enter the land and plant various kinds of fruit trees, you are to regard its fruit as forbidden — for three years it will be forbidden to you and not eaten.

In the fourth year all its fruit will be holy, for praising Yahweh.

But in the fifth year you may eat its fruit, so that it will produce even more for you; I am Yahweh your Creator. —Leviticus 19:23-25

Our last item on Yahweh's plan of what not to eat is the observance of His, set appointed times. Yahweh gives us instructions for when not to harvest any crops. Unless one is growing his own food, it would be hard to know exactly when that time might be. However, the health point remains that every certain number of years we shall eat less than during previous years.

Yahweh calls it a rest for the land in the Scriptures, but it is also a rest for the body. Both of these scriptures above and below confirm Yahweh has a plan and a schedule. According to the Scriptures, He will bless you if you obey them with the highest-quality foods in the ideal amounts and on His timing.

Sabbath Rest

Six years you will sow your field; six years you will prune your grapevines and gather their produce.

But in the seventh year is to be a Shabbat of complete rest for the land, a Shabbat for your Creator; you will neither sow your field nor prune your grapevines.

You are not to harvest what grows by itself from the seeds left by your previous harvest, and you are not to gather the grapes of your untended vine; it is to be a year of complete rest for the land.

But what the land produces during the year of Shabbat will be food for all of you — you, your servant, your maid, your employee, anyone living near you. —Leviticus 25:3-6

It has now been revealed to you what foods are taboo according to Yahweh. If you looked at most people's diets, you would see that many of the things they shouldn't be consuming are part of their typical diets. I was the same way until I learned the truth. If you didn't know, you had no reason to change. But now that you know, what are you going to do?

Their delight is in Yahweh's Torah; on his Torah they meditate day and night. —Psalms 1:2

Chapter 15: How We Were Designed to Eat

FOOD COMBINING CHART

DO NOT EAT FRUIT WITH ANY OTHER FOOD EXCEPT GREEN NON-STARCHY VEGETABLES

ACID FRUIT
Blackberries, Pineapple, Grapefruit, Raspberries, Lemon, Strawberries, Lime, Tangerines, Orange, Tomatoes*
[Eat before other fruits]

SUB-ACID FRUIT
Apple, Fresh Fig, Papaya, Apricot, Grapes, Peach, Blueberries, Kiwi, Pear, Cherimoya, Mango, Plums, Cherries, Nectarine

SWEET FRUIT
Bananas, Dates, Dried Fruit, Thompson & Muscat Grapes, Persimmon, Raisins

MELON
Cantaloupe, Honey Dew, Casaba, Persian, Crane, Sharlyn, Crenshaw, Watermelon
[Eat with no other fruit]

CARBOHYDRATES
Soaked and sprouted beans
Soaked and sprouted grains
Squash**
[Not recommended: cooked beans, grains, grain products, potatoes, squash and yams]

OILY FRUIT
Avocado
[A superior source of essential fatty acids]

PROTEINS
Coconut, Olives**, Nuts, Seeds
[Not recommended: beef, butter, cheese, eggs, fish, fowl, milk, pork, soybeans, yogurt]

NON-STARCHY VEGETABLES
Asparagus, Chard, Green Beans**, Spinach
Broccoli, Collard, Kale, Sweet pepper**
Brussels Sprouts, Cucumber**, Kohl-rabi, Turnips
Cabbage, Eggplant**, Lettuce, Zucchini**
Celery, Endive, Parsley

MILDLY STARCHY VEGETABLES
Artichokes, Beets, Carrots, Cauliflower, Corn**, Peas**

IRRITANTS - USE SPARINGLY
Garlic, Leeks, Onions, Radishes, Scallions, Shallots

Carbohydrates ↔ Sweet Fruit: POOR
Carbohydrates ↔ Non-Starchy Vegetables: EXCELLENT
Oily Fruit ↔ Carbohydrates: GOOD
Oily Fruit ↔ Proteins: POOR
Oily Fruit ↔ Non-Starchy Vegetables: EXCELLENT
Proteins ↔ Non-Starchy Vegetables: EXCELLENT
Proteins ↔ Carbohydrates: POOR

* Tomatoes only combine with non-starchy vegetables, seeds, nuts, olives, avocados, cucumbers and sweet peppers.

** Botanically classified as a fruit, but its biochemical composition places it in a non-fruit food combining category.

Chart compliments of Dave Klein

CHAPTER 16

When We Were Designed to Eat: There Is a Time for Every Purpose under the Sun

There can be a way which seems right to a person, but at its end are the ways of death. —Proverbs 14:12

Whenever I hear a discussion or lecture about eating according to the Scriptures, the debate or topic usually ends up being about vegetarian vs. meat eating. In my opinion, too much time is spent on this one issue and not enough on the more important topics. The Scriptures clearly address all matters concerning diet, including the meat-eating debate. However, people seem less focused on other issues that have a far greater significance. From a health standpoint, if people gave as much attention to being obedient to Yahweh's designed eating schedule as they do about what foods are acceptable, there would be far fewer believers suffering from disease.

> *The ten horns are ten kings who will come from this kingdom. After them another king will arise, different from the earlier ones; he will subdue three kings.*
>
> *He will speak against the Most High and oppress His saints and try to change the <u>set times and the laws</u>. The saints will be handed over to him for a time, times, and half a time.* —Daniel 7:24-25 [NIV]

Believers have become so distant from Yahweh's designed eating patterns that they practically live opposite from the manner He intended. Nearly everyone eats for incorrect reasons, at improper times, and way too much. This may seem like a bombshell to many people, but eating three meals a day was not the standard. Neither were the five or six meals that have become the norm today.

People seek to appease their pleasures, paying little attention to the dreadful consequences that follow. In addition, they disregard their surroundings and atmosphere when eating. They eat while stressful emotions rage up inside them, making it nearly impossible for their bodies to easily digest their meals. Eating lots of meals throughout the day also stresses the digestive tract, because it does not allow the previous meal proper time to fully digest. After all this, they wonder why they are not healthy.

Yahweh's Schedule

There is a time for everything, and a season for every activity under heaven. —Ecclesiastes 3:1 [NIV]

We have been designed to be on schedule! Our magnificent Creator Yahweh has given us all the required instruments, along with the intelligence to comprehend the perfect schedule for us to enjoy healthy, long, satisfying lives. If we want to be in the best of health possible, it is essential we live on this schedule.

The Start of the Day

According to the Scriptures, the beginning of day starts when the sun goes down and our night-light (the moon) rises. Yes, the evening is the beginning of the day! This seems incredibly unusual because our man-made clocks and modern time teach us the day starts at midnight.

The information I reveal in this book can only result in successful, healthy living if we stop listening to man's calendar and clock and start to obey the appointed dates and times Yahweh has revealed to us in His Scriptures. The sooner you phase out living according to the schedule of man and begin observing the schedule our Creator planned for you, the better off you will be.

Unlike man, who saves the best for last, Yahweh gives us the best and most important first. Sleep is the most essential ingredient for our health that we require, but we often become deficient in it. Good, proper sleep is so valuable to our health that Yahweh planned it to be the very first act each day in our daily schedule. When His night-light (the moon) appears, it's time to rest and sleep. During resting and sleeping, our bodies cleanse, heal and rebuild. It's very common today that people do not get enough sleep. More common is they do not sleep at the right times. By departing from Yahweh's schedule, we are destroying our health. If you do not adhere to Yahweh's intended sleeping patterns, it will be nearly impossible to follow His eating schedule.

Time to Go to Sleep

To determine the perfect time to be sleeping according to Yahweh's schedule, it is imperative to keep in mind the sun and moon are Yahweh's designed method of telling time, as opposed to the clock on your wall. We may need that clock on the wall to schedule business meetings and live in the world, but remember, it is instrument of this world. If you want to have supreme health and energy, it is best to get in the habit of revolving your life around Yahweh's clock as much as possible.

According to Yahweh's plan, the healthiest time to go to sleep is at the beginning of the day: sundown or soon after. Because the majority of the world revolve their lives around man-made clocks, this is nearly impossible nowadays, especially during the months when the days are shorter. However, we should still attempt to wind down our days and go to sleep not too many hours after sunset, the sooner the better.

In Yahweh's design, the days are usually shorter during the colder months for a reason. During the colder climate, the body usually is more stressed than during the warmer months. In addition, the foods of the winter season are commonly denser than summer foods, so more energy will be used to digest the heavier foods. The increase in work and stress would require more rest and sleep. The nights are longer during these months, giving us a sign to sleep more.

The foods of the warmer months and climate are less dense. They have more liquid and digest more easily. Because of this, we require less sleep during the summer months. The days are longer and nights shorter during these months, again setting a great model to plan our sleeping and eating schedules around.

The geographical location where a person lives can sometimes create an issue observing Yahweh's clock: for instance, you may live in Alaska, where the sun never sets during the summer months, and it is always light outside. This doesn't mean we can eat all night and that there is no ideal time to sleep. Of course, in those situations you would have to make adjustments. As man continues to drift farther from his natural environment than he was intended to reside, the harder but more important it is to be wise about Yahweh's schedule. I would suggest praying about it first in those situations, but remember: wherever you live, sleeping between the hours of 9 p.m. and 5 a.m. is usually best and what Yahweh intended.

Instead of arranging to go to sleep at sundown, the majority of people nowadays have just begun preparing to eat their biggest meal of the day after sunset when it is dark outside. In addition, they make plans to go out for entertainment after they eat. They do not comprehend that once the sun goes down and the moon appears, the rhythm of the body slows down. Eating just prior going to sleep or anytime when it is dark outside is quite out of synchrony with Yahweh's schedule and never recommended. Even eating five hours before sleeping is not suggested. If people really understood how unhealthful it is to consume any food when it is dark outside or within five hours of going to sleep, they would be more careful to avoid it.

Eating right before going to sleep is not good because the body is digesting food well after the meal is eaten, sometimes up to five hours after! When the body should be resting but is digesting your last meal instead, your sleep and health suffer. You may go to bed at one time and appear to be getting needed rest, but what is really taking place is digestion for the first five hours instead of the important cleansing that normally takes place during sleep. Even if you stay in bed with your eyes closed for eight hours, often only three hours of important, healing sleep has taken place. It's no wonder why the later people eat at night, the more tired they are in the morning.

Without man-made night-lights, we would rarely get an urge to eat when daylight disappears, and it is dark outside. Relaxing and sleeping would be our preferred activities. It is common these days for people to work a 9 a.m. to 5 p.m. job. It would be a healthy habit if people became accustomed to sleeping from 9 p.m. to 5 a.m. This is the ideal time period for sleeping, because during this time of night, the body does the most cleansing if it doesn't have to use energy on digesting food.

On the topic of sleep, a general error often made is that people are inclined to concentrate on the amount and not the quality. The number of hours is important, but more significant is the quality of sleep. There are four different stages of sleep, and it is during the last stage that deep healing and cleansing are taking place. It is common today for many people to reach this level-four stage of sleep only briefly during their sleeping hours. Although they have been in bed with their eyes closed for 6 or 8 hours, they toss and turn all night. Even though they spent a good amount of time in bed, they are not well rested in the morning. Observing Yahweh's set eating and sleeping plans will establish the greatest opportunity to get the optimal amount of deep, stage-four sleep.

Besides not eating late at night in order to assist the body in obtaining more deep, stage-four sleep, some other good tips would be not to watch television or work on the computer at least three hours before going to sleep. As opposed to how people often feel, work is stimulating and so is viewing images on a screen. Some people believe the sound of a television helps them fall asleep, but it usually keeps them up later than if they didn't watch it. What usually makes them fall asleep is the high-fat snack they are eating while watching late-night television. Studies show gluttony makes people drowsy, similar to alcoholism. People can actually get drunk from eating too much.

Stimulation is the body's built-in response to danger. However, overstimulation can create exhaustion of the adrenal glands and overuse of other hormones and various organs of the body. But the worst result of stimulation is that it keeps people from being obedient to Yahweh's timetable. Stimulation prior to going to bed will make it nearly impossible to get to sleep at the intended time.

Relaxing before going to sleep, or "winding down" as we refer to it, is the best way to assure a good night's rest: not only relaxation of the outer body, but also the internal organs of the body. An empty digestive tract creates relaxation throughout the body. Another good way to relax the whole body and mind before retiring if the weather is nice outside is to take a pleasant walk. Also try listening to some classical music. The best way is to read the Scriptures and pray.

It is believed that drinking water before going to sleep is a good idea, but I disagree. I suggest not drinking any water or liquid at least two or three hours before going to sleep. Drinking within of few hours of retiring for the night wakes us up throughout the night to go to the bathroom. Each time you awaken during the night, you are taking yourself out of the deep, stage-four sleep your body requires. If you follow Yahweh's schedule and diet, you should have had enough water throughout the day (which is important) such that you are not thirsty at night. You will be well hydrated if you drink enough water throughout the day.

Good health requires we get a certain amount of sleep each night. Arising early in the morning while still getting the necessary amount of sleep can happen only when we get to bed several hours before midnight.

Ideal Time to Awaken

Awakening at the appropriate time (at sunrise) helps you obtain important sleep and rest while preparing you to be refreshed and ready to do your daily activities when you arise. Today's man is often too tired to get out of bed early in the morning hours due to late-night eating and retiring well after the midnight hour. Because of work and other daily activities, people are usually forced to awaken well before their bodies have completed the job of cleansing that takes place during the deep stages of sleep.

Lack of sleep is one of the prime causes of sickness. The majority of people do not get enough sleep because they overeat. The more a person eats, the more sleep he requires, because more cleansing has to take place. So overeating makes it much more challenging to follow Yahweh's time schedule.

Nature is the perfect model for us to learn Yahweh's plan.

Take the sunrise for instance. The transition period each day from darkness to daylight does not happen immediately. There is an adjustment period from the first gleam of light along the horizon before the sun fully rises. The body also needs time to awaken and adjust each morning. Stimulating it too quickly can be injurious to your health.

Eating too soon after waking is not healthy because it stimulates the body and does not provide enough time to adjust naturally to the next phase of the day. When you arise at 7 or 8 a.m., there is usually not enough time before starting work to adjust from nighttime to daytime. This is another reason waking around 5 or 6 a.m. is a wiser time to choose. If you are eating according to Yahweh's timetable, it will give the body several hours to adjust before eating your first meal.

We must stick to His schedule to be healthy. We should arise refreshed and ready to start our work at least at sunrise and maybe even a few hours before sunrise every day. Again, this may seem like an impossible task, but results reveal all around the world that people who awaken before or at sunrise (without an alarm clock) usually have better health and live longer.

Lazybones! How long will you lie there in bed? When will you get up from your sleep? —Proverbs 6:9

Other than nocturnal animals, just about every other creature and animal in nature gets up at or right before sunrise unless sick or diseased. The birds start chirping, the flowers begin to open, and the air is the freshest it will be all day. Life truly seems to awaken all around upon sunrise. Similar to sick animals, only sick and diseased people will awaken well after sunrise.

Some people claim they are "night" people or "not morning" people. In the Scriptures, Yahweh's people were always morning people. The enemy is always lurking about, but it is in the darkness and the late-night hours we become most tempted. Sure, we can be a light in the darkness. If you are preaching in front of a bar at 3 a.m. in the morning for people to repent and listen to Yahweh, this is wonderful! But most people out and about at that time are usually pleasing the enemy more than they are pleasing Yahweh.

People commit the sin of overeating and overindulgence in all things more often at night than during the day. Not that this doesn't often happen during the day also, but just pass most restaurants at nighttime, and notice that they are much more crowded than in the daylight hours. After the sun goes down, it seems our guard also goes down, and we are more tempted during the night hours than the day hours.

The most important part at being successful and sticking to Yahweh's time schedule is getting to sleep early so you can awaken early. If you awaken too late in the day, your whole schedule will be off.

A lazy person is as bad as someone who destroys things.
—Proverbs 18:9 [NLT]

If you do not get the required amount of deep sleep, you will be tired and lazy. When you become lazy, you no longer have the energy to achieve the schedule Yahweh has planned for you. A person with no energy is usually too lazy to even accomplish the things he needs to get done, let alone do the things he has no motivation to do. Laziness also shows a lack of interest or priority. When your first priority is to stay up late to see who won the ballgame or American Idol, Yahweh's plan is not that important on your list of things to do. My point is, when we are lazy, we usually are not eager to stick to a schedule.

We usually have no problem arising early when we are excited about our day's plans. Take a woman on her wedding day. No matter what time she gets to sleep, she rises extra early on her wedding day with excitement, making sure everything is done and ready. If she has planned well, she most likely will get to sleep early the night before so she is well rested in the morning to start her busy and exciting day. She knows she has a schedule to follow, and she does her best to prepare to be on time! We should all be just as excited and prepared every moment of our lives to make sure Yahweh's planned schedule for us goes as smoothly as possible.

Let's look at some examples from Scripture of people who were up early every morning, ready and excited to live according to Yahweh's schedule. If my writings don't inspire you to get to bed earlier so you can wake up early and refreshed, hopefully these people's examples will. We need to utilize our energy and resources wisely.

Abraham got up early in the morning. —Genesis 19:27

Jacob got up early in the morning. —Genesis 28:18

And Yahweh said to Moses, Rise up early in the morning.
—Exodus 8:20

And Yahweh said to Moses, "Get up early in the morning."
—Exodus 9:13

And Moses wrote all the words of Yahweh. He rose up early in the morning. —Exodus 24:4

Samuel got up early in the morning. —1 Samuel 15:12

David got up early in the morning. —1 Samuel 17:20

Honoring Yahweh's set schedule is like a revolving circle. The more you adhere to Yahweh's sleeping schedule, the more practical it will be to eat according to the pattern He designed for health. On the other hand, the more obedient you are with keeping the set mealtimes, the easier it is to comply with His sleeping times.

Now that you know the problem, solving it is another issue. Many people are very addicted to a certain way of doing things. Even at the cost of their own health, some are not willing to change their ways. They get themselves used to living unhealthfully, and they cannot seem to leave their comfort zones. They don't want to change their diets, don't want to stop watching television, don't want to get on an exercise program, etc. They are simply addicted more to the harmful things than they are in faith.

If you want to be healthy, you have to believe in Yahweh's schedule and live *it*. Rise each day early so you can start each day at the planned time. If you have a plan to get up at 6 a.m. to exercise, eat a nice breakfast at 7 a.m., and so on, but wake up late in the day instead, there goes your plan.

People today overwork and undersleep! A good sign of this is the need for an alarm clock to get out of bed, and the need for coffee or some other drug to stimulate the body once we are up. The amount of sleep each person needs is different for everyone based on health status, diet, age, and many other lifestyle factors. If you need coffee or an alarm clock, there is a good chance you are not getting enough sleep.

Trust Yahweh! He will supply all your needs. If sleep and rest is something we all love to do, why do we cut it short each morning? Many people will answer that they have to get up and go to work. That is fine, but did you ever notice that when your work is your passion, you make sure you get enough rest to do a good job the next day? We get up with much energy and excitement to get the job done, but when we do not really like our jobs, we can barely get out of bed in the morning.

The job we have can be a big factor in the amount of attention we put into our plan of getting enough rest. We all have different lifestyles and different tasks to get done each day. We know how many hours we have each day to achieve our goals. Based on our needs, it is very helpful to plan our days wisely. Yahweh has important jobs for each of us, and He has helped us plan our times to give us the ultimate schedule to achieve all our goals.

While we are talking about being obedient to Yahweh's planned times for us, I cannot leave out information about Yahweh's weekly, monthly, and yearly plans for our well-being. Just as Yahweh gives us a daily schedule to follow, He also designed other appointed times for us to observe. Most so-called believers have no clue that the Scriptures talk about these other appointed times that are for their well-being.

I urge each person reading this book to search the Scriptures about Yahweh's weekly Sabbath, monthly new moon, and spring and fall feast days, such as Passover, Yom Kippur, and Tabernacles.

Many have been deceived to believe these days do not benefit them, but Yahweh says of course they do. Being blessed with a weekly Sabbath rest, a monthly new-moon rest, and yearly set-apart times of rest will help you see Yahweh's plans more clearly for the present and future times. No matter where we are in the world, if we obey Yahweh's guide, we will be blessed.

The following text I found in a great book called *The Entering Wedge*. It is used with permission. I could have rewritten it in my own words, but it is so well put and such a good message that few people consider.

The Summer Diet and the Winter Diet

As Yahweh caused vegetation to grow in the summer and to be dormant in the winter, He consequently constituted man to thrive on fresh garden produce during the summer and on dry during the winter. The fact that no tree can survive the summer without its leaves, but that it does well without them during the winter, again points out that a human being cannot fare well if he neglects to make his diet of fresh garden produce when in season, but that he can fare splendidly on dry winter foodstuffs when the fresh are out of season.

Moreover, as Yahweh did not from the beginning provide present-day transportation facilities, did not make it possible for man to import or to export foodstuffs from one remote locality to another, He constituted him to thrive best on the things which his own locality or the one closest to it can produce. To him, therefore, all foods grown elsewhere become secondary, and those which are not in season he does not need. In other words, while the fresh produce is the best for one's health in the summer, the dry is the best for him in the winter, unless he lives where the fresh produce naturally grows during the winter months too.

From these considerations, one can logically conclude that the person who lives in a warm climate needs to eat more of the fresh foods, but a person who lives in a cold climate needs to eat more of the dry, preserved, concentrated, heat-producing foods. He who does otherwise is, as it were, firing his house furnace full blast in the summer and running his house cooling system full blast in the winter! Is it not a wonder that a man thus tampering with his body can long survive through it all? If a deciduous tree should, were it possible, shed its leaves in the summer, or put them on in the winter, it would never have a chance again to try such an off-season idea.

In pre-engine transportation times, only a "ruler" could obtain out-of-season foodstuffs: strawberries, cherries, etc., when the snow flurries covered the trees and the icicles spanned from the roof to the ground.

Having this in mind, Inspiration warned, "When thou sittest to eat with a ruler, consider diligently what is before thee: and put a knife to thy throat, if thou be a man given to appetite. Be not desirous of his dainties: for they are deceitful meat" (Proverbs 23:1-3).

In Solomon's time, only a ruler could have used the numerous dainties made from white flour, refined sugar, and other commercial foods, but modern machinery now brings the ruler's "meat" to everybody's table, and consequently the modernized world is feeding on "deceitful meat," meat that does not supply the body's needs, that does as much good to men as a fisherman's bait on a hook and line does to a fish that goes after it.

Fruit is a summer food designed to keep the body cool and moreover, it is more of a dessert than a meal.

Canning of foodstuffs has become another health-destroying device, because the majority of people try to subsist on canned goods the year around. If you wish a prosperous and happy life, then break away from artificial, lawless life and thus from the world's ills.

CHAPTER 17

Set Times to Eat: Yahweh Separated the Day from the Night for a Reason

The information in this chapter has been paraphrased from author Doug Mitchell's article "The 'I'm Being Religious about Eating' Diet." You can view the entire article at www.the-branch.org.

> *Then to the crowds Yeshua said, "When you see a cloud-bank rising in the west, at once you say that a rainstorm is coming;*
>
> *and when the wind is from the south, you say there will be a heat wave, and there is.*
>
> *Hypocrites! You know how to interpret the appearance of the earth and the sky — how is it that you don't know how to interpret this present time?"* —Luke 12:54-56

The Scriptures reveal the ideal times for us to consume our food. Just like all topics, it has taken man thousands of years later to reveal by research what the Scriptures told us long ago was best for us. But still, even though the evidence is out that eating late at night is not healthful, people still do it. They are completely addicted. When you have Yahweh and science showing the same evidence, and you still go against the information, there is a very good chance you are being controlled by the enemy.

The most common issue people have pertaining to diet is that they eat too late into the night. Eating too often throughout the day is another widespread issue, but late-night eating is the major dilemma. There is absolutely no other sinful action committed daily as often as this form of gluttony. It is physically and spiritually unhealthy and completely against Yahweh's plan. This may seem like too strong of a statement, but when you realize gluttony of food and/or drink leads to every other sin, you will agree.

One question I get often is, "How much and how often should we eat?" As stated in this book, the amount of nourishment each person requires will vary depending on many factors, but today most people are eating a lot more than they need to be. How often we should eat is another issue altogether.

People are consuming too many meals too often, and it's another reason their health suffers. With good study of Scripture, we can see how Yahweh's chosen people consumed only two meals a day at certain specific times. Health teachers now are agreeing that these times would be the most ideal times to consume our food. The Scriptures show us the connection between consuming food and the customary times of worship as found in the Scriptures: the third and ninth hours of the natural day, which correspond to about 9:00 a.m. and 3:00 p.m.

> *They are headed for destruction! Their god is the belly; they are proud of what they ought to be ashamed of, since they are concerned about the things of the world.* —Philippians 3:19

We can see the connection today between the massive number of daily meals that people are eating and the lack of worship, lack of knowledge, and failure to give thanks to Yahweh for our food. As people lost connection with Yahweh, they looked toward food as their comfort. Emotional eating and idolizing our foods can get us sick very quickly, and this is what is happening on a daily basis.

I have been studying health for many years, and can confirm all these facts with scientific evidence. However, even people who have never studied the topic would agree the systems and organs of the body are more efficient in digestion of food when the sun is out, and we don't overeat. I can't stress enough how important it is to eat, sleep, and rise according to the times Yahweh suggests are best for us. Once you wake up either with a lack of needed rest or too late in the day, the whole schedule is thrown into havoc.

Natural Time

Yahweh said, "Let there be lights in the dome of the sky to divide the day from the night; let them be for signs, seasons, days, and years."
—Genesis 1:14

Yahweh made the two great lights — the larger light to rule the day and the smaller light to rule the night — and the stars.
—Genesis 1:16

Yeshua answered, "Aren't there twelve hours of daylight?"
—John 11:9

At the time that He said this, the people of the world had a number of ways of keeping time. The scriptural method of keeping time uses sunrise as the beginning of the first hour and sunset as the end of the twelfth. This means that as the seasons change and the days become longer and shorter, the hours would likewise become longer and shorter necessarily.

Yahweh's people of old were told not to learn the customs of the nations around them, who were sun worshipers in one form or another (Deuteronomy 18:9). As far back as ancient Babylon, men were devising ways to measure hours of equal lengths. Water clocks, sand clocks, and many others were invented. In the 11th century A.D., an Arab astronomer even developed a sundial that would read in equal-length hours. Yet Yahweh's faithful people used none of these as the rule to establish their hours of worship and thus their mealtimes. When they were faithful, they retained nature's health laws by receiving spiritual and physical nourishment in a timely manner.

The third and ninth hours, which were used for the services in the earthly sanctuary, varied in length seasonally. Why didn't Yahweh give His people a method of measuring equal-length hours if it would have been beneficial to them? The one who was to "think to change times and laws" (Daniel 7:25) didn't stop with trying to change the Sabbath or the feast days or the months and years, but he has extended his reach even to the hours of the day, thereby affecting the hours of worship, eating, and sleeping by this attack on nature's Author.

Today, many health researchers are rediscovering that the human body is directly affected by the sunrise and sunset. The period in between is referred to as the photo-period. They have been finding that the big experiment of living by the clock rather than by the sun is not really best for any natural being. They are also reaching the same conclusion about the staying up late at night made possible by electrical lighting. There has always been a temptation to unnecessarily "burn the midnight oil."

There are conflicts with nature that arise when one eats at the same hours by the clock. In North America in the winter, there are only around 10 sixty-minute hours of daylight. In the summer, there are around 15 sixty-minute hours. If one is in the habit of eating supper at 6:00 p.m. each day, said meal would be taken after sunset in winter, a practice which is contrary to good health, as will be explained later.

Perhaps the greatest testimony against the use of equal-length hours is the need for Daylight Saving Time, which was incorporated to compensate for the extra energy used to artificially illuminate the hours when the work hours were out of sync with the day's light. Twice a year, those people of the earth who take their meals by the clock and go on and off Daylight Saving Time by adding or losing an hour of a day throw off their entire bodily cycles and bring an unnecessary shock to their systems. It takes some people months to recover from the change in mealtimes, and no one who follows the practice of eating by the clock (rather than by the sun) is immune from a certain amount of trauma due to the drastic changes.

The purpose of this chapter is to aid us in being restored to our natural cycles and to the ensuing health and well-being.

As we have discussed already, divine time can be based only on the sun and moon. It is best when eating to have the same mealtimes each day, but that does not mean eating at the same clock times each day. The times of the sunrise and sunset change each day, so 9 a.m. today on a man-made clock is not the exact time as 9 a.m. tomorrow. According to Yahweh's schedule as revealed by the sun and moon, each day has a different length. The man-made clock never takes this into consideration, and this is where the major confusion happens.

Regardless what the man-made clock shows, the only way to figure out the same time each day is to start counting from sunrise. Every annual rhythm of nature calculates time in this manner. Plants, ocean waves, and even animals live their entire lives according to the sun and moon.

For instance, plants open and close their flowers at the same times each day. No matter how much we talk to them and tell them what to do and not do, they have coded within them that they are designed to respond to nature's factors and set times. The times of their patterns may change each season based on factors like the climate during the time of year or other natural occurrences, but the seasonal times will always be the same as long as plants are left in their natural environments.

However, if you take plants out of their natural environments without mimicking those environments, the plants will die. For them to have any chance of survival, you would have to continuously supply them with a close approximation to what they would naturally receive for their existence. The first and last sign that something is wrong is that they are no longer on their natural schedules.

If you can find a way to move a plant to another otherwise compatible environment but keep its life on the same needed schedule, it will survive. However, it will not thrive as it would in its natural elements. The further you take something away from its natural element, and the longer you keep it away, the lesser the quality of life it will produce.

Florists have figured out how to keep plants alive by doing a good job of imitating their original environments. Zookeepers do an excellent job of creating an environment for each animal from all over the world to mimic its natural environment. Even buying a goldfish and bringing it to your house in a fish tank provides a decent job of creating a similar environment for the animals.

Man can find ways to mimic the sunlight and the rain by way of florescent lights and watering to keep plants on their correct schedules. He will cut and build a forest area for animal enclosures and will spend time and money on a beautiful fish tank to duplicate the beauty of the ocean floors, but he cannot manage to keep his own body on its correct, natural schedule. He certainly has the capability to do it; he just chooses not to.

To figure out the best times for us to consume our food and how often we should eat, we can look at yet another sign from Yahweh. Every natural function of nature — the water, the atmosphere, and even the earth — has two cycles. Within each, the daylight and the nighttime, there is a high and low tide. These tides are based on forces of nature that astonishingly man has figured out, but yet ignores the data regarding his own body.

These tides of nature work in harmony with our own bodily rhythms. Tides reveal the ideal times for sleeping, eating, cleansing, and being active. The further we stray from these times, the more stress we put on our bodies to stay healthy. Just as plants will survive in a mimicked environment and new schedule, so can we thanks to the amazing power built within us by Yahweh. Man has an amazing power to adapt; however, each time we do something off schedule, it is shortening our lives and making us sick in the process.

Understand that if you give a plant the right food at the right times and keep it in the best environment for its type, it will last much longer. Today, everyone is looking to avoid sickness and live a long life, spending lots of time and money searching for antiaging secrets. From growing many sprouts, I have noticed there is a science to getting the freshest, biggest, most tasty, and nutritious sprouts. That science is all the factors mentioned in this book, but it all comes down to keeping it on its designed schedule.

Eating according to the Body's Schedule

Woe to you, land, when your king is a child, and your leaders start their parties in the morning!

Happy are you, land, when your king is well-born, and your princes eat at the proper time, in order to stay strong, not to get drunk!
—Ecclesiastes 10:16-17

Wisdom of old has also spoken of the consequences of eating

Chapter 17: Set Times to Eat: Yahweh Separated the Day from the Night for a Reason

at the wrong times.

Where photo-periods are concerned, the natural process is still the same no matter what we eat. Our digestion slows down significantly after the sun goes down and doesn't quicken again until the sun rises. Those who eat a large meal near or after sundown will usually have the feeling that they are not yet finished digesting it when they rise in the morning, even though it may have been 8-12 hours since they ate. This feeling may last an hour or two after rising.

This slowdown in digestion is attributed to the increase of melatonin, which is a major factor in restful sleep. Large meals eaten near or after sundown never really get the full assimilation which is possible and end up robbing the body of its fully refreshing sleep, because the digestive system is still trying to do its major work during a time when it should be at rest. Yet when the same type of meal is eaten earlier in the day, the body is wide awake and able to complete its work without interfering with the cycles of rest because of the activity of the day and the effects of the daylight.

This one factor alone of eating large meals towards the end of, or after, the daylight hours is the major reason why many people's biological clocks are on a 25-hour cycle rather than on a 24-hour cycle. Forcing the body to try to digest a heavy meal during the time that its digestive processes are slowed, due to the sun's having gone down, extends the actual time for the complete digestion of the food and the cycling and replenishing of the digestive juices, and thus ends up overlapping with the time when the breakfast is usually taken.

Eating after the sun goes down, often only a few hours before going to sleep for the night, causes a poor night's rest due to a working digestive tract, with the resulting need for more energy to finish the digestion of the unprocessed load in the system from the late meal. The practice of putting new food on top of that which is not finished digesting causes fermentation in the digestive system and creates gases and toxins that injure the system and need to pass out of the body through the elimination organs — the skin, lungs, kidneys, liver, and bowels — thus unnecessarily burdening them and causing unpleasant odors, gases, skin conditions, constipation, and other ailments.

The destructive practice of taking late meals is made worse by taking an early, heavy breakfast. As the digestive system has not completed its work on the previous night's meal when another large meal is put into it, it is forced to work overtime without its necessary rest and rejuvenation time, thus robbing the system of more needed energy. This also tends to make one's mental and physical powers sluggish and dull in the early hours of the day. Then the early, heavy breakfast is usually followed by an equally heavy lunch and similar supper.

So not only is the body strained by all of the work involved in the continuous processing of food, but the overabundance thereof is converted into fat or is passed along in a semi-digested state, thereby causing other maladies.

Researchers have observed that when more food is taken only a few hours after eating, something from the food already in the first part of the intestines is ejected from there, even though it has not yet gone through its full processing. As the body doesn't want to expel the contents of the intestines in a semi-digested state, the taking of more food before the previous amount is fully processed causes that previous mass to be impacted together with the mass which preceded it, thereby causing a stretching of the intestines, the creation of unwanted gases and toxins, and a delay in the normal elimination time (constipation).

It simply makes sense that one should have as many eliminations as meals, but such is rarely the case when people eat three or more meals per day. Researchers have noted that when someone eats a piece of fudge only two hours after eating a meal, the elimination is pushed back four hours. If another piece is taken after just another two hours, the elimination is pushed back eight hours. And so the problem compounds exponentially.

The best time to consume food is when the body is naturally in its digestive rhythm. There are two times a day this happens. These would be third hour and the ninth hour of daylight. These two times are the ideal times to consume our meals each day. Eating when it is dark outside is the worst time to eat.

Eating during the third and ninth hour of daylight may seem unusual because it is not the customary eating times. In addition, it is only two times a day as opposed to the traditional three meals per day. We have strayed so far that we don't even eat three meals a day anymore, now consuming many meals and snacks all day long. As long as the quality of the food is very high, two meals a day should be sufficient for our nutritional needs. Eating many meals throughout the day, whether big or small, never lets our system digest its last meal and rest. It also takes us off of Yahweh's planned schedule.

Snacking or eating between meals is not part of Yahweh's schedule: two meals a day at the appointed times are. If the third and ninth hours of daylight are the ideal times to eat our meals, you can now begin to understand why getting to bed and rising at the correct times becomes so vital.

Pagan traditions of sun and moon worship are partly the reason why our culture has adopted eating three times a day: upon sunrise, when the sun at its highest peak, and at sunset — also on full moons and other pagan-celebrated feasts. In the Scriptures, we see the Jewish nation giving daily sacrifices during third and ninth hours of each day. The people all ate after the daily sacrifices, two times each day to make sacrifices to Yahweh at the temple. (Animals were sacrificed and eaten by the priest afterward. We will discuss the issue of eating meat later.)

The animal sacrifice has been done away with, since the blood of our Messiah has redeemed us for our sins. We no longer require animal sacrifices, but the times and actions of a sacrifice are still important for us to keep today. Before eating at the ideal times, we should still make a sacrifice and praise Yahweh before we consume our meal. I suggest sacrificing your most valuable asset, your time. Before you eat, open your Scriptures and read a proverb and sing a psalm to Yahweh.

The only time in Scripture that eating at nighttime took place amongst Yahweh's chosen people was during the last supper. This was certainly a set-apart night out of the norm. If you must, it is okay to occasionally take a break from the norm for a special occasion, but it's what usually follows the majority of the time that will determine the quality of your life. I do find it interesting that during the night of the last supper, three of Yeshua's followers could not stay awake while He went to pray in the garden (Matthew 26:40). Possibly they were so full from the food and lack of digestion because of eating at nighttime that they couldn't keep their eyes open.

When Exactly Is the Third and Ninth Hour of Daylight?

> *Yeshua answered, "Aren't there twelve hours of daylight?*
> —John 11:9

Two meals a day were usually served in Israel during the time the Scriptures were written. Other nations did not follow this model and suffered for it.

> *He said, "If you will listen intently to the voice of Yahweh your Creator, do what He considers right, pay attention to His Torah, and observe His laws, I will not afflict you with any of the diseases I brought on the Egyptians; because I am Yahweh your healer."*
> —Exodus 15:26

Up to now I've mentioned the third and ninth hours of daylight are the best times to eat your meals. By the man-made clock, the 3rd hour usually starts between 7 a.m. and 9 a.m. for our first meal, and the 9th hour starts between 2 p.m. and 4 p.m. for our second meal.

Because Yahweh's timetable begins and is calculated by a different method, you are really not eating at a different phase of the day because no matter what the man-made clock says, you will always be eating during the 3rd and 9th hours of daylight.

Some health books suggest certain mealtimes but never take into account that Yahweh's times are decided by the sun and moon. So for instance, eating at 7 a.m. every day could make it light outside in one season and dark the next. As suggested, it's never good to eat when it's dark outside. The wonderful news about Yahweh's eating pattern is that it will always be light when eating. Yahweh never changes, and we can still follow His divine plan for the ideal times to eat.

> *The ravens brought him bread and meat in the morning, and bread and meat in the evening; and he drank from the stream.*
> —1 Kings 17:6

So two times a day is the ideal number of meals we should eat. What is also notable is that after fire had come down from heaven and consumed Elijah's offering on Mt. Carmel at the time of the evening sacrifice, he told King Ahab, "Get thee up, eat, and drink" (1 Kings 18:41) [KJV].

Then after Ahab had that evening meal, Elijah told him, "Prepare thy chariot, and get thee down, that the rain stop thee not. And it came to pass in the meanwhile, that the heaven was black with clouds and wind, and there was a great rain. And Ahab rode, and went to Jezreel. And the hand of Yahweh was on Elijah; and he girded up his loins and ran before Ahab to the entrance of Jezreel" (1 Kings 18:44-46).

So that evening meal, right after the evening sacrifice, was still early enough in the day (before sundown) to allow them to prepare Ahab's chariot and ride a fair distance before night fell.

The Third and Ninth Hours

Because nature calculates time by a different method, you are really not eating at a different phase of the day. No matter what the man-made clock says, you will always be eating during the third and ninth hours of daylight.

The correct, specific time for your two meals, of course, will always depend on the season and the time of sunrise where you live. It may already be light out at 7 a.m. in the summer but dark at 7 a.m. in the winter where you live. It's never good to eat when it's dark outside; wait two hours after sunrise, no matter what the season or where you happen to be, and you will be eating your first meal at the optimal time.

There is a helpful website where you can just input the times of sunset and sunrise where you are, and it will tell you the times of the third and ninth hours: www.the-branch.org. (You can also download a spreadsheet from that website that will help you figure out the times each day.) In case you are not able to get online every day, here is how to figure it out:

There are 12 hours in the daytime and 12 hours in the night. However, we must not assume there are always 60 minutes in an hour. That is a man-made idea. Only near the equator are the lengths of the day and night periods almost equal. The times of the sunrise and sunset determine how long an hour truly is. Anywhere else in the world, that is always changing. In the winter, there are more hours of darkness, and in the summer, more light. So how do you tell what the true third hour and ninth hours are?

Find out from a calendar, a weather website, a newspaper, or an almanac the times of sunrise and sunset. Once you have those times, the rest is easy to figure out. Here's an example:

- Suppose sunrise is 6 a.m., and sunset is 6 p.m. The third hour of daylight would start at 8 a.m., and the ninth hour would begin at 2 p.m.
- Now, for a more complicated example, suppose sunrise was 6:33 a.m. and sunset 8:17 p.m.:
- 12 hours = 720 minutes (if there were 60 minutes to the hour)
- Add any "extra" minutes, in other words, any minutes exceeding 720 minutes. From 6:33 a.m. to 8:17 p.m. is 13 hours, 47 minutes, or 104 extra minutes.
- Add 720 + 104 = 824 minutes
- Divide 824 by 12 to get the "true" total minutes in an hour, 68 minutes (in this example)
- Starting from the time of sunrise, use 68 minutes for each hour to calculate the beginning of the third and ninth hours, as in this example:
- 6:33 a.m. + 68 + 68 = 8:49 a.m., which is the beginning of the third hour
- 6:33 a.m.+ 68 + 68 + 68 + 68 + 68 + 68 + 68 + 68= 3:37 p.m., the beginning of the ninth hour
- If you choose to eat 3 meals a day, eat the first a little earlier and the last meal a little later, and add one meal in the middle.

We Are All in Diverse Situations

Each person is in a different situation, and the condition of one's own body is never identical to anyone else's, so you have to pay attention and give your own body the attention it needs, not based on what everyone else is doing, but based on what it requires. Yahweh planned for us to all live according to the same divine schedule. No matter our situation, the plan does not adjust to it. We have to alter our circumstances to fit His divine plan for our lives. No matter how different the state of our health may be, there is a universally ideal time to consume our food. Just like every rhythm of life, the time never changes based on how we feel or on when Daylight Saving Time may be according to man-made clocks. The immortal times never change.

However, the conditions of our bodies are at different stages, due to how we have treated them in the past. Where an individual is concerned, the amount of vitality he has or lack of it will determine the exact type of diet he requires. We each require different amounts and types of food. A sick person lacking nutrients will need a much different food plan than a healthy person who has been eating a good diet for many years. No matter what the state of your body and the history of your diet, you deserve the best quality food for your particular situation. We will talk more later about the quality of food, but keep in mind the best times to eat those foods are the same for everyone.

Even though we have all been designed to keep the same eating and sleeping pattern for ideal health, we each have different chores and jobs each day during our lives. For some of us, switching our eating and sleeping patterns will be simple because we have a lot of free time to do so. For others, it may not be as easy due to our hectic lifestyles. For instance, a single person with no job will have a much easier time than a big family where both parents are working. Sometimes our jobs may not coincide with Yahweh's schedule.

It takes time to adjust, and depending on the positions we are in, some of us may be able to adjust sooner than others. We each have to decide for ourselves what is truly feasible and what we are just doing out of habit. If your family is all in the habit of eating dinner around 8 p.m. every night, that's not a healthy habit. However, if everyone is working till 7 p.m., it may not be feasible at the present time to eat together before 8 p.m. This does not make it wise to live against Yahweh's schedule just because we have a good excuse to do so. If Yahweh truly wanted each of us to live according to His timetable, and if you asked Him in prayer to show you how, He will reveal the answer.

A good practical adjustment to the above situation may be instead of the family eating together for dinner, they can have their first meal of the day together if it is important to them to sit and enjoy a meal together. Most people working later into the evening usually start their day later, so instead of each person eating breakfast at different times and eating dinner together, maybe you can all eat breakfast together and take a late lunch at your jobs by yourself and enjoy your last meal of the day at a healthier time.

Using Common Sense

> But not all foods wholesome in themselves are equally suited to our needs under all circumstances. Care should be taken in the selection of food. Our diet should be suited to the season, to the climate in which we live, and to the occupation we follow. Some foods that are adapted for use at one season or in one climate are not suited to another. So there are different foods best suited for persons in different occupations. Often food that can be used with benefit by those engaged in hard physical labor is unsuitable for persons of sedentary pursuits or intense mental application. Yahweh has given us an ample variety of healthful foods, and each person should choose from it the things that experience and sound judgment prove to be best suited to his own necessities.
>
> —*Ministry of Healing*, pp. 296-297.

I do not expect everyone to be able to switch his schedule and change his habits overnight. Some of you may decide never to change, but we can all make some adjustments to help. Some suggestions may be—

- No longer eating anything after dinner. After-dinner eating or drinking is an unhealthful but common habit.

- Going for a walk in the morning instead of just popping out of bed and right into the kitchen for a meal.

It's very important we evaluate our own situations, but even more important that we consider what Yahweh designed our bodies for and to do our best to stick to that plan. When we each became believers, we gladly adjusted our lifestyles to please Yahweh. Many new believers had to make radical changes, but joyfully did so. We all have choices. If our passion is to please Him, even those times where it seems impossible, with faith we will thrive.

Lastly in His important schedule, Yahweh provided us with certain daily, weekly, monthly, and yearly times of rest, not only rest from our daily jobs, but complete rest from all our physically draining chores of everyday life.

The majority of believers completely ignore these orders within Yahweh's commands and keep working away as if they mean nothing. Some believers understand the importance of the commands and are obedient to cease from work on these special days. However, just about every believer views rest as sleep or relaxation, never taking into account that the most work the body will ever have to do is done during the process of digestion.

Every bite of food a person consumes makes the body work hard using much energy. The lower the quality of food, the harder the body's digestive system works, and the more food consumed, the more energy is required. Very few people realize you are not giving the body the true rest Yahweh requires when you are eating too much food. For this reason, it is wise to eat less food, less often during these special commanded times of rest.

These times are not only for rest, but also for fellowship and worship with Yahweh, to enjoy Yahweh's presence without any other distractions, including thinking about food. The cleaner we are in the inside, the easier it is to be in connection and communication with Yahweh.

This is why fasting and praying is so powerful in the Bible. Whether it is eating fewer meals these special days than on normal days or just eating less during each meal, Yahweh gave us these resting times for our benefit, and we should stick to His timetable for when it is best to do so. These rests from eating can assist the body in the annual healing and cleansing it often needs while also giving it rest from the consistent energy drain eating causes.

I believe the Sabbath (Friday sundown to Saturday sundown) is an ideal day to consume less than the amount usual on other days. There are some current health teachers who say they have seen research to confirm the most healing time for the body is on the Sabbath. If this is true, eating less on this day would assist the body in healing, but more importantly, it would give the digestive system a well-needed rest each week. A day when most people eat and move around the most, Yahweh said rest and move around the least. See how we have transgressed from His plan?

This book is about health according to the Scriptures; however, it is important to mention that man once again changed Yahweh's Sabbath day from Saturday to Sunday. This change is one of the many steps taking man away from Yahweh's divine schedule.

Some readers may be wondering about fasting (not eating food) completely. There is only one day in Yahweh's plan that commands us to fast (Yom Kippur), but there are many other scriptures regarding fasting. I believe fasting is very beneficial if done with wisdom. It helps give the body ultimate rest, and there is no greater time to communicate with our Creator than during a fast. This is why fasting and praying work so well together. Not eating for a day every once in a while is very helpful for healing and cleansing. It is also a wonderful way to break an addiction to overeating.

An important lesson I've learned about fasting according to Yahweh: It's not the same as, "I was just so busy I didn't have time to eat." Anyone can easily occupy his time that he misses a few meals, but it's quiet time with Yahweh when we get the benefit.

Some people choose to go on a longer fast for more than

just one day. I do not believe the length of a fast should ever be scheduled. Whether a short fast of one or two days or a longer fast, we should stop the fast when the body responds it is time or when Yahweh tells us. I've seen too many people lose the benefits of fasting by stating before the fast how long they are going to fast. Three important keys to successful fasting if longer than one day are—

1. Make sure you are getting complete rest. If it is not possible to take off from work and chores, it may be wiser to do a fresh juice diet instead of fasting.
2. Do not proclaim your fast to the world. Fasting should be a personal journey between you and Yahweh — and sometimes your close family members.
3. When ending a fast, eat less than you normally would have eaten for a few days afterwards. There is a tendency to overeat after spending several days of not eating, but this is very harmful and usually wipes away all the benefits of the fast.

Once you experience and enjoy this cleansing, healing, resting time, you will be inspired to eat less more often. Whatever you decide, keep in mind it is in Yahweh's schedule that we take a break at some point from eating.

I have attempted to cover as much as I can about the dangers of overeating in this chapter about consuming too many meals too often, and also in previous chapters about eating too much food in those meals. I have been teaching for years that two of the biggest causes of disease from a physical standpoint are overeating and undersleeping and the connection they have with each other.

Then I started to teach the real cause of our self-inflicted disease: not obeying Yahweh's Word or even worse, going directly against it. I am so thrilled to find Doug's website that has many more great articles about the daily times to have our meals and also a great chart to figure out when the 3rd and 9th hours start each day, no matter what season we are in. I am even more excited to see the example set in Scripture about the daily times to give thanks to Yahweh before our meals.

The information about diet is beneficial, but we cannot receive any benefit from the food unless we properly glorify Yahweh. Even if you are strict in the quality of your food, do you glorify Yahweh and thank Him for your food? We move so fast today, making time for everyone except the One we should be making time for the most. Why do so many people miss this important message?

Those who place so much food upon the stomach, and thus load down nature, could not appreciate the truth if they heard it. They could not arouse the benumbed sensibilities of the brain to realize the value of the atonement and the great sacrifice that has been made for fallen man. It is impossible for such to appreciate the great, the precious, and the exceedingly rich reward that is in reserve for the faithful overcomers. The animal part of our nature should never be left to govern the moral and intellectual.

I am thankful for this information, and I will waste no time putting it to good use. I pray everyone will search this information out and experience the benefit and blessings that come from being obedient and thankful to Yahweh each day.

Here is some more great text with permission from *The Entering Wedge*.

Work and Rest, Year Round

Time, we know, is divided into two parts, night and day. In the summer (the season for raising and gathering the supplies for the winter months), the days are long, but during the winter (the season in which there is no farming to be done), the nights are long. These Divine regulations definitely suggest that one should put longer hours in working during the summer months than he should during the winter months. And how long should they be? — evidently as long as the sunlight lasts. Yes, the parable of Matthew 20:1-17, too, plainly declares that Yahweh commanded His servants to start early and work through to the end of the day, to sunset.

So while the natural way of life demands longer working hours during the summer months, it demands shorter working hours during

Chapter 17: Set Times to Eat: Yahweh Separated the Day from the Night for a Reason

the winter months — a daily average year round of 12 hours' work and 12 hours' rest. One who complies with all the requirements which Truth herein recommends complies with the natural laws of his being, with the laws which promote good health and which bring happiness into the home. But if he disregards these laws, he cannot of course expect to receive more than his investment permits. And too, a person should clearly see that the full amount of work is just as essential to good health as is the full amount of rest, that one should balance the other; and that to the extent he violates these laws, just to that extent will he suffer the penalty they impose. "Because thou hast...eaten of the tree," again warns the Creator, "...in the sweat of thy face shalt thou eat bread till thou return unto the ground" (Genesis 3:17-19).

Think of the unnatural life the world is now living! It endeavors to get along on as little work and rest and on as much fun and play as possible. It eats denatured and out-of-season foods, drinks alcoholic, spirituous, and drug-containing liquids all day long — what a swill! A wonder that it still lives! Indeed, it is "wretched, and miserable, and poor, and blind, and naked"; and not knowing its condition, it says, "I am rich and increased with goods, and have need of nothing!"

Recap

- 2 meals a day
- 3rd hour and 9th hour
- Don't eat at night
- Rest and cleanse the body

Yahweh's Vision vs. Television

And if your eye causes you to sin, gouge it out and throw it away. It is better for you to enter life with one eye than to have two eyes and be thrown into the fire of hell. —Matthew 18:9 [NIV]

Up to this point, I'm doing my best to make it clear that Yahweh has given us a schedule to follow. I will give you information in future chapters about exactly what foods are best to eat according to the Scriptures, but since it is so common that people eat at the wrong times due to being led away from Yahweh's schedule, I have to warn every reader of the most common trick of the enemy to get people off of Yahweh's schedule. It's your television set. If you have already figured this out and do not watch television or spend only a very little amount of time viewing it, I'm sure you can agree that nothing saps our time and energy more than television programming. In addition, nothing keeps us as far away from Yahweh's schedule as television does.

In chapter three, I began by saying people use man-made clocks to control people's lives today. The hands on the clock seem to dictate where you should be and what time you need to be there. I suggested we need to observe Yahweh's clock much more carefully. Nowadays, cable and networks have become our new clocks. People schedule their entire lives around their favorite shows on television. They call it programming for a reason: that's what the advertisers are doing to you.

The name alone, "tell-a-vision," shows us it's just a box that tells us about visions. The mind control through scientific machinery and human mind manipulation being told today on the tell-a-vision is not a healthy message, and it's certainly not of Yahweh.

Not only do we attempt to enjoy these messages, but we also allow our children to experience these harmful images. What the eyes absorb can easily become part of our lives. Mentally, it brainwashes us. Yahweh tells us to love the things He loves and hate the things He hates. Television programming flips that around. Spiritually, it keeps us from finding time to spend with Yahweh and understanding and believing his Word. And physically it makes us lazy.

Chapter 17: Set Times to Eat: Yahweh Separated the Day from the Night for a Reason

Did you know there is a reason why it's called programming? Because it is programming you to be on their schedule instead of Yahweh's schedule. This book is not about the negative effects of television, so I won't get into the all the facts, but the more time people spend watching television programming, the more overweight, sick, and depressed they become. We live during a time now when people spend more hours than ever before watching it. We also live during a time when there is more disease than ever before. See the connection?

I'm not suggesting the television set is harming you, although it might be. It's what people are watching that's doing the real damage. A good example is when people suggest "money is the root of all evil." No, it's not; it's what people do with the money. So the television set is not the issue; it's what's being viewed. I suggest only watching DVDs, because we can control what we see and when we see it.

The programming advertisers know how to trick you. If you don't believe that, just ask yourself why they would spend 10 million dollars for a 30-second commercial during the Super Bowl. I would say 90% of the shows on television today consist of messages that go against what Scriptures say. Even when you view a righteous show, the commercials are usually not. Advertisers understand human thinking and know how to get people to overeat. The most common thing that keeps people awake later than they should be is television.

Television is one of the things in our comfort zone that people think they can't live without. You can certainly live without a television in your life. In fact, the quality of your life would improve. The best thing would be not to have one in the house if you are too tempted to view it, but you are on the right track if you can at least limit it to DVDs only.

I could go on and on about the harmful effects of television that far outweigh any (if any) positive reasons to have one, but the main question to ask yourself is, is this television bringing me closer to know Yahweh? Or is it taking so much time from my life that I don't have time to pray, read my Scriptures, and find more ways to glorify our Heavenly Father?

My suggestion is to get rid of your television and replace the time you spend watching television with reading the Word of Yahweh. If you desire, you can still enjoy DVDs on your computer and even download quality movies and television shows.

One of the best sites I have found is www.glc.us.com. This site is based on a satellite television station that airs wonderful shows and interviews with Torah teachers. There are many new wonderful websites, videos, and films to enjoy if you strongly desire to spend much of your time in front of a screen. Just be careful not to make them an idol in your life and to view them at the right times according to Yahweh's schedule.

PART 4
Whom Do You Worship?

CHAPTER 18

We Make an Idol Out of Our Food:
No One Is Able to Serve Two Masters.

They are headed for destruction! Their god is the belly; they are proud of what they ought to be ashamed of, since they are concerned about the things of the world. —Philippians 3:19

There is no area or topic where people sin more than in making an idol out of their food. Each time the average person sits down to eat to satisfy his tastebuds, appetite, or habit, he is putting his own pleasures before Yahweh's needs. This is breaking the Second Commandment that says you shall have no other idols in your life. People treat their food like a god, worshiping it.

The pleasure of the taste and smells of food and drink have taken precedence over giving pleasure to Yahweh. It has become the number one idol in people's lives. Drink is not limited to alcohol. Many believers today consume many different beverages simply for pleasure: coffee, soda, energy drinks, etc.

The only pleasure that we are to enjoy, according to the Scriptures, is to please Yahweh by following His Torah. When we go against them, no matter how good it makes us feel, we are breaking the Second Commandment, making an idol out of whatever is giving us the pleasure.

When we make food more important than Yahweh, we are in big danger. Many so-called righteous people wonder why they are sick. They spend much time giving praises to Yahweh, but as soon as they see some type of good-looking food, Yahweh becomes second place in their lives.

Even if we can manage not to make food more important than Yahweh, we should still not have food as an idol. The simple fact that we overeat so much shows how much of an idol we have made it. If people had Yahweh on their hearts and minds as much as they do their next meal, there would be much less need for prayer for healing of disease in the churches and assemblies.

One of the powerful reasons for fasting when seeking Yahweh's Word is that it takes our focus off food and puts it on Yahweh. When is the last time you fasted or went a whole day with no food? Did you miss the food? When is the last time you went a day without reading Yahweh's Word? Did you miss it as much as you missed the food?

When we make an idol out of our food, we break the First and Second Commandments. A great scripture that talks about how people made an idol out of their food is found in Nehemiah. And it shows also how people suffered for it. Today we commit and suffer for this same sin.

> *So the children went in and possessed the land, as You subdued ahead of them the Kena'ani* [Canaanites] *living in the land, and handed them over to them, along with their kings and the peoples of the land, for them to do with as they wished.*
>
> *They took fortified cities and fertile land, possessed houses full of all kinds of good things, dug-out cisterns, vineyards, olive groves, fruit trees in plenty; so they ate their fill and grew robust, luxuriating in Your great goodness.*
>
> *Yet they disobeyed and rebelled against You, throwing Your Torah behind their backs. They killed Your prophets for warning them that they should return to You and committed other gross provocations.*
> —Nehemiah 9:24-26

The situation in this scripture passage is no different from today. People are disobedient and rebel against Yahweh and Torah. They reject and kill His prophets, and today people are more obese than ever. On a daily basis they commit great wickedness. And then they wonder why so many are sick today.

The Torah is the so-called meat of the Scriptures; everything else in Scripture after the Torah is examples and stories of how we should treasure Yahweh, listen to His Word, obey His guide, and be thankful for it. Without the Torah, we would not know what is good or evil. There would be nothing to be our standard. Once we get away from the guide of Yahweh as found in the Torah, man will just use his own feelings as his guide, with no standard, and he will just do what is right in his own eyes and not Yahweh's. Most people today have never read the whole Torah, and most so-called believers do not follow it. And people are suffering because of that.

There are many examples in the Scriptures of people who were righteous and followed the instructions of Yahweh's Torah. We should take these examples as our true role models in life. Just think about how our world would be different if everyone followed the Word of Yahweh.

Yeshua as Role Model

The greatest example of an obedient Torah observer is Yeshua Himself. This is why many refer to Yeshua as The Living Torah. The whole basis of the Scriptures is supposed to be the covenant between Yahweh and man. Our side of the deal is that we have to want to please Yahweh. As a gift to make it easy to do that, Yahweh gives us the guide, Torah, telling us how to please Him. Man has grossly overlooked this guide, so Yahweh sent His Son Yeshua as a living example of how to have a heart for the Torah. Even before Yeshua came, there were some righteous men who didn't overlook the guide of the Torah and who did their best to follow it.

Moses as Role Model

The first person who comes to mind is Moses. Moses was one who didn't have a strong passion to lead under his own will: he knew that pleasing Yahweh was more important than pleasing himself. He put his own needs under Yahweh's desires. Moses didn't want to be a leader, but he accepted that role when Yahweh made it clear to him that he was the chosen one to lead the Israelites out of Egypt and reveal the Torah to them.

Moses finally accepted the job not because he felt like he wanted to do it, but because pleasing Yahweh was more important to him than pleasing himself. Recall that during a time when many people were living to around only 80 years old, Moses made it all the way to 120. Pleasing Yahweh and putting Yahweh first while trusting in His plan for us will help us to receive the blessings He has in store for us.

Noah as Role Model

Another great righteous person in Scripture was Noah. Noah also wanted to please Yahweh, so he put Yahweh's desires ahead of his own. Noah listened to Yahweh without any protest, and this pleased Yahweh. We can be righteous and listen to Yahweh like Noah, but many people waste time and blessings struggling with Yahweh's Word like Moses. Moses finally listened to Yahweh and accepted the role of being the person to free the Hebrews out of bondage in Egypt, but at first he protested. He didn't immediately agree as Noah did.

It's fine and righteous to follow His Word, but we have to learn to be more like Noah. When we hear Yahweh speaking to us, we have to react positively and not protest. Not only did Noah jump when Yahweh spoke, he was also sure to always put Yahweh's desires ahead of his own. Like in Noah's times, there aren't many people today who are willing to do this. This is the reason why Yahweh said about Noah—

> *For I have seen that you alone in this generation are righteous before Me.* —Genesis 7:1

Noah was grateful for Yahweh's love toward him, and he showed it. The way to express love for Yahweh during the time of Noah was to sacrifice a clean animal. Realizing how blessed he and his family were to be spared of Yahweh's wrath, the first thing Noah did after getting off the boat was to make not one, but many, sacrifices to Yahweh.

> *Noah built an altar to Yahweh. Then he took from every clean animal and every clean bird, and he offered burnt offerings on the altar.* —Genesis 8:20

Noah listened, obeyed, and was thankful. If we want to be healthy, that's the answer right there.

Listen

Yahweh is always speaking to us, either through Scripture or however else He decides to get His message across to us; but because of so many distractions in today's world, we don't hear Him.

Obey

Many people choose not to listen because they know that if they did listen, then they would have to face the decision whether or not to obey. We are trained in this world to be selfish and to disobey. Some people may read this and get offended, especially believers with sincere hearts. Many ministers today do not teach us to obey Yahweh's Word. They use grace as an excuse to disobey.

Be Thankful

It's one thing to hear what Yahweh wants and obey, but to do it with joy and pleasure is also important to our health. Many people struggle with doing Yahweh's will and do it only because they feel they have to. We shouldn't do anything out of a sense that we "have to," but because we want to. This is what Paul was talking about when he said that the Torah should not enslave us; it should free us. The greatest sign that we feel good about doing something is to show thanks. It's hard to be thankful for something you didn't like or that you feel provided nothing of value to you.

Noah understood that Yahweh made man to be a tiller of the soil and to be a caretaker of the land. Therefore, the second thing Noah did after leaving the ark was plant a vineyard.

Noah, a farmer, was the first to plant a vineyard. —Genesis 9:20

Noah put Yahweh's desires first and took care of his own future needs second. In Noah's eyes, Yahweh's desires took precedence over what his fleshly human nature would want. Noah's needs were simply to listen, obey, give thanks to Yahweh, and live according to His Word.

Job as Role Model

Another righteous, obedient man of Scripture was Job. Job pleased Yahweh fully and put Yahweh's desires before his own needs.

My favorite scripture is one by Job, a man who always kept focused on Yahweh as number one in his life no matter what happened. Most people today seem to worship the things of this world, especially the things that seem to keep them alive. But we see in this verse below that Job says Yahweh's instructions are so important that they are even more than his necessary food.

> *But He knows the way that I take; When He has tested me, I shall come forth as gold.*
>
> *My foot has held fast to His steps; I have kept His way and not turned aside.*
>
> *I have not departed from the commandment of His lips; I have treasured the words of His mouth more than my necessary food.*
> —Job 23:10-12 [NKJV]

The word 'necessary' is such an important part to that scripture. It is one thing to say I can forget a meal or two and fast for a few days, but to honor Yahweh's Word above food that is necessary is to say His instructions are more important than my physical life. We just don't find people with a passion and desire for Yahweh's Word like this today.

Of course, Yahweh does not want us to harm our bodies and starve for Him. He supplies all we need when we truly need it. However, He wants us to look at everything He gives us as a blessing or a gift and not take it for granted. When it comes to food, that's what most people do.

We have to be like Daniel. He put his life on the line to be obedient.

Do we see the importance of these examples? Anyone who knows Scripture can see how Yeshua, Moses, Noah, Job, and many other righteous followers of Yahweh upheld the Torah as the most important thing in their lives as their standard to please Yahweh. Regardless of the trials these righteous people went though, they found joy in pleasing Yahweh. It is so important for us to reject the world's view and standards and always be faithful to the guide of Yahweh.

This whole topic can be covered in Psalms 119. The writer of Psalms 119 tells us of praising Yahweh and the importance of a truly faithful life to Yahweh and His ways for us, as opposed to a faithless person's life.

In the Scriptures, there are examples of what the result will be when we live against Yahweh's guide and set our own personal needs before pleasing Yahweh and living according to his standards. We have to take joy in Yahweh's guides just like the writer of Psalms 119.

In summary, Psalms 119 basically says—

Blessed are those who live by the instructions of Yahweh and observe His witnesses.

Blessed are those who seek Him with all their heart and do no unrighteousness.

Blessed are those who diligently guard His suggestions and are never ashamed of them.

Blessed are those who delightedly follow the wisdom of Yahweh's instructions and continue to keep learning about them.

Blessed are those who have chosen the way of Yahweh's righteous guide and joyfully meditate on it every day.

Do you want to be blessed? Sickness is not a blessing; it's a curse. Disease is not what Yahweh wants for us. Open your Scriptures to Psalms 119, and see exactly what Yahweh wants from us.

Yahweh understands that in the flesh we are weak and struggle, and for this He gives us mercy. However, He is also jealous, angry, hurt, and upset when we are obedient to other elohim and reject His words and warnings. Along with His great mercy also comes great anger. If we go against His Word too often, we will suffer for it — not because He wants to harm us, but because rejection of His Word puts us in danger.

The greatest thing Yahweh gives us is the ability to choose to obey. If we didn't have this ability as an option that we can choose, but instead we were forced to obey, then we would be just like robots following His Word. Even then, under those circumstances, the world would be much better off, but the key to our relationship with Yahweh is to please Him. And nothing pleases him more than our choosing to follow His guide not because we have to, but because we want to.

What Do the Scriptures Say about This Sin of Making an Idol Out of Our Food, and How Harmful It Can Be?

You are not to make for yourselves a carved image or any kind of representation of anything in heaven above, on the earth beneath or in the water below the shoreline. —Deuteronomy 5:8

History shows Yahweh is not happy when we make an idol out of our food. Two times in Scripture Yahweh destroyed the people because of their corrupt living and wicked sins. These are two outstanding instances when most people didn't want to please Yahweh. They gave all of their hearts to other elohim and put their own pleasures before Yahweh's. They suffered drastically for their disobedience.

These two instances were the times of Noah and the times of Lot. In both these instances, people were living so far against Yahweh's guide that He ended their existence, one time with a flood and the other time with fire and brimstone from heaven. It is interesting to see that in the midst of all their sins and disobedience, the most common sin during both these times was eating against the guide Yahweh gave them, against His Torah, or instructions.

Just as in both those times, man today has gotten so far away from Yahweh's Torah that because of it, disease and sickness are everywhere. Yeshua warns us that because of our mass sin, the same drastic result experienced during the times of Noah and Lot will be cast out upon us as well.

Chapter 18: We Make an Idol Out of Our Food: No One Is Able to Serve Two Masters

Do not follow the crowd when it does what is wrong.
—Exodus 23:2

There is more to it than just the mass number of sins they committed on a daily basis. Both times, there was something the people of both times had in common. They were eating and drinking against Yahweh's Torah.

The times are coming more and more today the way they were then. It is quite interesting that believers see so many of the common sins, and many scholars predict the end is near, based on the actions of the people today.

Many people who know Yahweh's Word clearly see the wrong and mass sin that was committed in those days and today as well. The Bible even states many of the sins: violence, corruption, homosexuality, adultery, prostitution, and many other sins that are also so common today. To make matters worse, many of these sins are being committed within the church. Many people who consider themselves believers in Yeshua have not repented for their lustful behavior and continue to practice the same evils they condemn.

For men like these are not serving our Master Yeshua the Messiah but their own belly. —Romans 16:18

Of all the acts being committed by people in and out of the church, the idolatry of food and drink leads the list. There is no doubt about this today. All you have to do is see how people to react around food and how it controls most of their desires. Their lustful bellies lead them to all sorts of other sinful behavior.

No one can dispute the harmful results of overdrinking, but did you know eating too much food could get you drunk? Studies now reveal eating too much animal meat can create a desire for animal-like behavior. Like wild dogs, we live in a world where every sexual abomination is on the minds of society today. We no-excuse people seek to use all our energies to transgress as far as possible from Yahweh's schedule and instructions, and idolatry of food and drink leads the way. It is the beginning to the end.

We see during the times of Noah and Lot many sins being

committed. Yeshua tells us the exact conditions in the scripture of Luke:

> *In the days of Noah, people ate and drank, and men and women married.*
>
> *Likewise, as it was in the time of Lot: people ate and drank, bought and sold, planted and built.* —Luke 17:27-28

Now, it is amazing that Yeshua does not talk about the often-mentioned sins that are so obvious to us as being sin. Instead, He talks about the simple, common things of everyday life, and the two that are at the top of the list in both cases are eating and drinking!

We have taken a simple daily blessing from Yahweh (nourishment) and turned it into daily sins. That is not a singular sin, but plural sins.

> *Also, at the time of the Son of Man, it will be just as it was at the time of Noah.*
>
> *People ate and drank, and men and women married, right up until the day Noah entered the ark; then the flood came and destroyed them all.*
>
> *Likewise, as it was in the time of Lot: people ate and drank, bought and sold, planted and built;*
>
> *but the day Lot left Sodom, fire and sulfur rained down from heaven and destroyed them all. That is how it will be on the day the Son of Man is revealed.* —Luke 17:26-30

The times are becoming more and more today the way they were then. There is violence, corruption, homosexuality, adultery, prostitution, and many other sins. However, in this passage from the book of Luke, Yeshua tells us the exact conditions that existed in those days.

> *People ate and drank, and men and women married, right up until the day Noah entered the ark; then the flood came and destroyed them all.*
>
> *Likewise, as it was in the time of Lot: people ate and drank, bought and sold, planted and built.* —Luke 17:27-28

Yeshua mentions the common things of everyday life at that time, and not the gross sins that the people were committing. And He says that these are going to be the conditions prevalent when He puts an end to the world.

What is the significance of Yeshua stressing this? Many scholars explain that Yeshua is simply saying that life will be going on as usual when He unexpectedly comes again. They say that is all that is implied when Yeshua mentions the people eating and drinking.

None of these things are sinful in themselves, but they had come to be most important in those people's lives. These things came to be idols in their hearts. They had come to be gods to them. Most of these things are absolutely essential or quite necessary to us just to stay alive. But we need to keep our guards up and make sure we don't let this happen to us, making these things more essential than our relationship with Yahweh.

You can now hopefully see how living life a little against Yahweh's Torah will lead to doing it more and more. The first time we stray we may realize something is not right. But the more we get used to it and comfortable living in sin, the more it gets very dangerous because we end up living against Torah without realizing it; or we do realize it, but it's too much of a challenge to change.

As stated at the beginning of this book, the Scriptures are a book of opposites! The opposite of following Torah is living in sin. We have a choice; we can choose one or the other, but we can't choose both. Many of us are living against the guide of Yahweh, especially when it comes to eating and drinking, and we suffer for it.

Yahweh wants us to be righteous in all we do. Yahweh sees our hearts. If our hearts are in the right place, Yahweh will lead us to joyfully follow His Torah, and that will be pleasing to him. The world sees our results as more important than our efforts, but Yahweh sees us and judges us in a much more righteous way. Keep the effort strong, learn what's pleasing to Yahweh, and do your best to achieve it.

We need to have faith not by what we see, but what we believe before seeing.

> *You're not looking for me because you saw miraculous signs, but because you ate the bread and had all you wanted!* —John 6:26

Like Job, we must seek His Word more than our necessary food. Daniel also put his life on the line to be obedient—

> *But Daniel resolved that he would not defile himself with the king's food or the wine he drank, so he asked the chief officer to be excused from defiling himself.* —Daniel 1:8

> *How blessed are those who reject the advice of the wicked, don't stand on the way of sinners or sit where scoffers sit!*
> *Their delight is in Yahweh's Torah; on His Torah they meditate day and night!* —Psalms 1:1-2

CHAPTER 19

Meeting Your Emotional Needs: Yahweh Hears the Cries of the Righteous

It is important in writing to keep the subject positive so the reading can be inspirational, but when we talk about the subject of eating according to Yahweh's instructions, it is hard to stay positive, because so many people have been deceived into following man's instructions instead of Yahweh's. This is a common reason why just as many people who profess they are believers suffer from the same amount of disease as people who do not.

The enemy will find a way to tear us down and break us. Once we get addicted to something that is not healthful for us, it seems we are trapped. Instead of just praying for healing of disease, we need to pray for wisdom to see our addictions and have the strength to overcome them. The Scriptures tell us we can do all things through Him who strengthens us, but we often do many things by him who deceives us.

> *Don't be conceited about your own wisdom; but fear Yahweh, and turn from evil.*
>
> *This will bring health to your body and give strength to your bones.*
> —Proverbs 3:7-8

Enthusiasm Makes the Difference!

It takes a lot of discipline to reverse the pattern of unhealthful eating habits, but we all have discipline for whatever it is we love. You just have to love being healthy more than the taste of what's making you unhealthy. Or you have to hate being sick more than limiting yourself. Either way, you can do it. When you have desire, knowledge becoming discipline is not an issue. But there is something else that makes the difference: enthusiasm!

For me it began with exercise. That's partly where it started, because that's where I learned to eat so much so often. I was always into exercise and researched what I had to do (legally) to become big and strong. Everything I could get my hands on told me to eat more. So I did. I ate and ate and ate.

What exercising itself taught me was the importance of having a schedule, and not just in the mind. Write it down! We have money budgets and time budgets. Well, why not a food schedule?

Someone once told me a money budget tells your money what to do instead of your money telling you what to do. Well, a food schedule can tell your body when to eat instead of your emotions telling you when to eat. If you put some schedules together, you can be free from the day-to-day stress in no time. The Excel spreadsheet on my computer has been put to good use, but you can make it happen even with just a pen and paper.

I eat very little now and also with wisdom. I didn't do it overnight. It took me many years to change, not because I had to take so long, not even because I wanted to; I just didn't know any better. It's like when I was working out, I didn't know much at first, but a good trainer helped me learn a lot and save a lot of time in the gym. Well, I've taken the time when it comes to eating healthfully and making the correct adjustments that will give the best results. Let this book be your trainer.

I wrote this book because I understand how it is to keep trying something without getting results for lack of knowledge. I also know how it is to live with disease. I know how it is to be addicted to eating late at night and other eating issues. I know what pain and suffering is like, but I also know how to overcome them. I'm here to help you. This book is here to help you. You can turn around and make the needed changes in the right direction.

I always reflect on how amazing the body is. We can abuse it so much, but still it will last and even return to a healthy state as long as we get rid of the things causing the issue.

Barring some tragic accident, we will all eventually fall to our unhealthful habits if we don't change our ways in the right direction. Just because the body can survive for a long time living unhealthily, that doesn't make it safe to do so.

CHAPTER 20

Dealing with People: Remove Me far from Vanity

Should we care what others around us eat?

I care for and love certain people. It's sad and frustrating to see others completely avoid, ignore, or twist Yahweh's instructions. I am aware of the harmful consequences that follow. I do my best to help people who make unwise choices, but people many times have to learn for themselves. Often the only thing we can do is pray for them. Do not take that lightly, because that means so much. What is even more frustrating than being able to help someone and that person not wanting it is people who think you are wrong and try to convince you to change your ways.

It is very unwise to even get into a discussion with people who have no knowledge about the subject at hand. For example, you can attempt to teach nonbelievers that Yahweh's ways are best; but if they do not agree, it would be foolish to argue with them. If they are not believers, chances are they do not know or understand scriptures.

An even more challenging issue is finding someone who thinks he really does know but is completely misled. It is these types of people I run into most often, Christians who think they are correct but couldn't be more off the mark. They have very little knowledge of the Scriptures, and their actions are not producing any fruit. To argue your point with a person like this is an energy drain, a waste of time, and a foolish action.

It is written in the Scriptures—

> *But avoid stupid controversies, genealogies, quarrels and fights about the Torah; because they are worthless and futile.* —Titus 3:9

Do not get involved in foolish and unprofitable arguments.

This does not mean we should refuse to study, discuss, and examine different interpretations of difficult biblical passages, but it's a warning against petty quarrels. As foolish arguments develop, it's best to turn the discussion back toward a helpful direction and politely excuse yourself. We should avoid false teachers, not even bothering to be involved in their foolish discussions. Our overreactions can sometimes give more attention to their points of view.

The more I tested eating two times a day and saw the benefits, the more I questioned how I was ever able to eat any more. Also, after not eating after 3 p.m. for only a short time, I couldn't even imagine eating later in the day, let alone late at nighttime. Yet why was I able to realize this while not many other people do?

The reaction from people was no surprise. My family already thought I was nuts because I ate a raw food, vegan diet. They are right in one respect: you are what you eat, and I did consume nuts. So dealing with their reactions wasn't too difficult, other than my dad's fears, thinking I was going to starve to death, or my brother's of not being able to hang out with me anymore, because the only time we seem to be able to do anything is when he invites me out to eat dinner.

The reactions from my friends weren't too bad. Most of them knew I was healthy, and it didn't surprise them that I found a new experiment to improve the quality of my health. They were supportive, but interested to learn more, just as the general health community was. I started a blog, giving updates to keep everyone informed.

To everyone's surprise, I didn't lose much weight and looked better than I ever had. My wife noticed the positive changes right away. I'll never forget when she told me the whites of my eyes were as clear as ivory. My hair was fuller, and I no longer had the dry scalp that I'd had for years. From a dietary standpoint, not eating late at night was part of the answer, but I'm sure avoiding sweet fruit was the other.

Of all the reactions I got, the biggest surprise and most joyful was from my wife. I thought she was going to have a fit when I announced to her I'm not going to eat after 3 p.m. No more going out to eat for dinner was what I thought I was going to hear. To my pleasant surprise, she was all for it. She jokingly said, "You already eat a boring diet, so fine."

I'm sure the books on my bed nightstand talking about the advantages had something to do with her willingness to give up the late night candlelight dinners. She must have peeked at a few of those books, because in a short time, she was willing to give it a try herself.

As for dealing with the general public, I have never found eating only certain foods has to be an issue to me. If I couldn't find something to eat, I just wouldn't. Not a big deal.

There are many reactions you will get from people, and there are many reasons not to do this. I do understand that we need to work and make a living. If you truly enjoy your job and your life, I don't expect or even suggest you change them. However, I tell everyone that no matter how well you eat, if you are going to a job every day that you do not enjoy, your health will suffer big time.

The ideal situation would be to do what you love for a living while at the same time being able to eat healthfully. There should be no other answer! However, we live in a world today that is so far from understanding the impact on health emotionally, socially, and physically that the norm has become a sad state.

I know people who make over a $100,000 a year but have no time to spend with their families. When someone can live on $25,000 a year and be healthy and happy, why does someone need $100,000 a year? It all comes down to the lifestyles we have become accustomed to. We must change our ways, and it starts with our thinking. There is nothing wrong with making $100,000 a year and owning a big house, but if you are doing it at the cost of your energy and health, it's time to reconsider what you do.

So my reaction to people's reactions is not controlled by their reactions. Look at the word re-action. It means we changed our actions based on the situation. Before you read this book, you didn't have the information presented herein. I pray, but don't expect, that everyone who reads this book will follow the no-dinner diet, but if I can just get you to rethink about some of the choices you have made and take a new action, one that will support your health, then the purpose of this book was successful.

Do It for Yahweh!

Why eat healthfully? Why take the time to learn what is best for you? Why invest in something so costly? Because Yahweh wants you to, that's why! If you don't want to make the effort and take the responsibility to improve the health you have, because you are satisfied where you are at, understand this: Yahweh doesn't want you to settle for anything but the best! You can have more health and energy! You can live your life in a more excellent way!

Each morning you wake up, your prayer to Yahweh should be the same prayer Dr. Bisci told me about: "Give me an amazing understanding about the human body and health, more than you have ever shown anyone before."

To start each day, your passion should be to do better than you did the day before, to keep moving forward and to yield the greatest profit in your health, joy, and your whole life!

I meet many caring, loving people who have such a passion to help others, but our first duty to help man and serve Yahweh is the investment we make in our own self-development. Every ability our Creator blesses us with should be cultivated to the highest degree of perfection, that we may do the greatest amount of good we are capable of.

To accomplish this, we must make a wise investment in our own emotional, mental, physical, and spiritual health and well-being. We should not settle for anything less. The more we settle, the more we suffer the consequences.

The good news today is that more people are interested in taking responsibility for their health than ever before. The rising cost of healthcare and mass obesity from higher-fat foods are motivating people to pay more attention to disease prevention instead of dealing with the effects later on. They may not be the best of reasons for people to wake up, but the important thing is that people are finally waking up. People now want to be healthy.

We all have the capability and opportunity to be the best we can be. Yahweh gave us His Son Yeshua to help us accomplish the goal and overcome adversity. For us to settle and accept anything less than what He wanted for us would be robbing Yahweh the honor due to Him.

One of the most powerful statements I ever read was from the great Christian health writer Ellen White: "A failure to care for the living machinery is an insult to the Creator. There are divinely appointed rules which if observed will keep human beings from disease and premature death."

Obviously people have not been listening. The prophet Isaiah tells us the earth suffers for the sins of its people because they have twisted Yahweh's instructions, violated His laws, and broken His everlasting covenant (Isaiah 24:5).

Yahweh designed us and also designed that manual for us to stay healthy. If we were simply to follow His guidelines and instructions, we would reap the blessings that follow. We are living in sin when are not feeding our bodies with the highest-quality food He designed for us. This disrespect for His design will lead to disease very quickly. We live during a time when there is more disease than ever before in the history of man. We are also living during a time where more people than ever before are living against the moral and physical guidelines Yahweh gave us. Can't you see the connection between the two?

Yeshua warned us that prior to His return conditions would exist very similar to those which preceded the flood. Eating and drinking would be carried to excess, and the world would be given up to pleasure. In today's world, men seek pride, power, and pleasure on a daily basis. Disease may be the outward result of this sin, but the inward result is an unfulfilled life.

Those who love Yahweh are satisfied always with what they have. Those who ignore Him are always focusing on what they don't have.

People are consuming foods in excess and destroying their very own temples, the bodies Yahweh designed for them. We must keep our temples clean if we want to be healthy. Even in today's dark world, Yahweh's light shines. With a little research and study, you can find everything you need to stay healthy. Yahweh is always providing for our needs as long as we search for the answers to them.

The enemy wants to see us destroy ourselves with our own folly, overstuffing ourselves with chemically made foods and then seeking a doctor to heal us from our foolish ways — or even worse, seeking other gods or religious systems of the world. The Scriptures tell us it is best to put confidence in Yahweh, not man (Psalms 118:8)! When you accept Yeshua as your Messiah, you are making a covenant with Yahweh, a promise that you will trust, obey, and follow His path always, no matter the situation.

We see a great example in Daniel, who was told he would be put to death if he didn't bow to other gods. Daniel not only refused to bow, but he also refused to defile his holy temple by eating unclean foods (Daniel 1:8). Daniel is a wonderful example of a man who was put though the worst trials a man can go though and still did not abandon Yahweh's ways.

Do not be deceived by popular, New Age healing techniques:

Open my eyes, so that I will see wonders from Your Torah.
—Psalms 119:18

Many New Age therapies claim to manipulate or diagnose energies and their flows. You must judge and show discernment, because many of these therapies are not of Yahweh. Yahweh has a plan for us, and as long as we make the right choices, He will provide us with all we need. He gives us the information to always make the right choices, and He makes it possible for us to heal because of our faith in Him.

Any therapy that talks about moving "energies" is usually not of Yahweh, and you should run as fast as you can from it. There is usually some type of occult, metaphysical, New Age twist tied to it. Some words you should be careful with are, for example—

Reiki, meridians, yoga, prana, kundalini, auras, crystals, Zen, gurus, Transcendental Meditation, horoscope, Higher Consciousness Movement, the human potential or development, new thought, Eastern mysticism, Eastern spirituality, enlightenment, paradigm shift, occultism, ancient wisdom, Age of Aquarius, holistic health movement, alignment, affirmation, transformation, reawakening, spiritual tools and paths, shifting, balancing energy, centering, decreeing, meditation, channeling, astral projection traveling, empowering, energies, initiations, invocations.

This does not mean everyone who uses these words is an occultist. Not everyone who wears a crystal is either, but it can be possible that he has some related views or practices.

And finally there's karma, the idea that you get what you give: Some people claim karma is a lesson taught by the Scriptures, but they couldn't be more wrong. First, to have good karma, you have to do "good deeds" for good people and bad things to people who do bad things. No one is perfect. What is good is determined not only by our outside actions, but by what is in our hearts. Yahweh sees our hearts, and only He knows our true intentions. We are blessed to have Yeshua in our lives to help us make the right choices.

Yeshua and His disciples encountered a blind beggar on the street. The question arose as to who had sinned to cause this blindness. The question reveals the bad theology that "bad" things happen to bad people. The Messiah dispels their simplistic view of human suffering by explaining that all the events in our lives are given to display the wonderful works of Yahweh. It then is up to us how we respond when "Yeshua passes by" (John 9:1-3).

PART 5

Healing according to the Scriptures

CHAPTER 21

Disease or Not Disease: Choose Life and You Shall Live!

Hear, O earth! I am going to bring disaster on this people; it is the consequence of their own way of thinking, for they pay no attention to My words; and as for My Torah, they reject it. —Jeremiah 6:19

Disease as we know it today is not what Yahweh had in mind for us in His original plan. Originally, we were not made to have disease in our lives. There are many examples in His Torah which show that as long as we follow His words, we will avoid many of the self-inflicted (i.e., within our control) diseases that overcome many today.

The wonderful book *The Entering Wedge* really sums this topic up nicely. I am very pleased to quote the following text about disease and its causes from *The Entering Wedge*.

As thy days, so shall thy strength be. —Deuteronomy 33:25 [KJV]

This scripture plainly reveals that Yahweh never intended for man to be sick or weak and to pass away before his days are full, but rather that he should retain strength commensurate with his age and die not of disease, but of ripe old age:

And this also is a sore evil, that in all points as he [the wicked] *came, so shall he go: and what profit hath he that hath laboured for the wind? All his days also he eateth in darkness, and he hath much sorrow and wrath with his sickness.* —Ecclesiastes 5:16, 17 [KJV]

Naturally those who go on living independently of Yahweh are not only committing wickedness, even though unconsciously, but are also laboring in vain. Furthermore, their eating in darkness, not having Divine light on the subject, causes them to eat food such as brings not strength, but sorrow, wrath, and sickness.

The Causes of Disease

Disease has been identified in three different categories: hereditary, communicative, and self-created (acquired). This being so then, there must be three kinds of sin, three laws to transgress. Two of these laws are found in the Decalogue (Exodus 20:3-17): The first prohibits sinning against Yahweh and the second against our fellow men. The third is the law of health, the law which forbids transgressing against our own bodies (Leviticus 11; Isaiah 66:16-17).

Plainly then, sinning against Yahweh brings in its wake a hereditary curse, the kind that passes from father to son "unto the third and fourth generation of them that hate Me" (Exodus 20:5), saith Yahweh. Sinning against our fellow men brings communicative diseases, shown in the fact that when Miriam sinned against her brother Moses, she was stricken with the contagious disease leprosy (Numbers 12). And, "Honour thy father and thy mother: that thy days may be long..." (Exodus 20:12).

So, "Whatsoever a man soweth, that shall he also reap" (Galatians 6:7). Thus it was that when Haman built the gallows upon which to hang Mordecai, he himself was hanged on them (Esther 7:9, 10). And when Daniel was unjustly cast into the lions' den, his enemies were devoured by the hungry beasts, but Daniel was spared (Daniel 6:16, 22, 24). Moreover, when the three Hebrews were cast into the fiery furnace, those who carried them were consumed by the flames, but the Hebrews came out unharmed (Daniel 3:21-23). Also, "He that leadeth into captivity shall go into captivity: he that killeth with the sword must be killed with the sword" (Revelation 13:10).

It is therefore a never-failing fact that if one molests his neighbor or intends to do so, the harm will fall on himself. If he harms his neighbor's children, his own children will suffer as a result.

The diseases which are not inherited the sinner himself creates by sinning against his own body. Sinning against a neighbor or against oneself, nevertheless, is indirectly sinning against Yahweh also.

What Should Everyone Know?

If one is suffering from a hereditary disease for which his parents, grandparents, or great grandparents alone are guilty, he is of course helpless to do much of anything in the line of complete recovery, be it by dieting or by using drugs. He may, however, be able to control the disease or even to overcome it by being strictly obedient to the laws of Yahweh, knowing that nothing in the world will effect a cure for such illness but prayer, if Yahweh's wisdom so decrees.

On the other hand, if one is suffering from a disease which has been communicated to him or that is communicative, due to one's sinning against his fellow men, then to remove the disease once and forever, he must repent of his sin and practice the golden rule: "All things whatsoever ye would that men should do to you, do ye even so to them" (Matthew 7:12).

But if the disease is neither hereditary nor communicative, then it must be self-created: acquired by oneself by violating the laws of health and by not living right in one respect or another.

The wise will then correct their habits of living to make sure that they do not sin against Yahweh or against their fellow men, that they sleep, breathe, eat, drink, and work correctly and religiously. If there is a cure at all, they will have it.

The cause of each type of disease having now been defined, the sufferer of any of the three kinds of diseases may without difficulty determine which one of the three laws he is transgressing and paying the penalty it imposes as a result. If he is afflicted with complications of diseases, though, he must be breaking all of Yahweh's laws. Let him henceforth quit sinning in any line if he expects to recover and stay well too.

Many diseases are wrongly classified as contagious. For example, tuberculosis is not actually communicable, for when one becomes infected with the disease, he can effect healing if he begins to live right while it is yet in its early stages. Obviously, then, if one always lives right, he need not fear of the disease ever getting a foothold in his body. So in the last analysis, a number of so-called contagious diseases are not such in reality. Strictly speaking, they are infections brought on by oneself. And now, how fortunate should one consider himself to know that right living and right doing, with faith in Yahweh, actually do away with a multitude of sorrows!

Summarizing the Causes of All Diseases

Those who wonder what is the cause of this, that, and the other disease may quickly test every case.

It is now fully understood that life and death are at war with each other as are the nations among themselves. One nation's army may pour fire upon another, but not all of the soldiers receive the same kind of wound, even though the whole army be under the same fire. In like manner, the bodies of men are the soldiers, and causing disease is the Enemy's mighty weapon in the warfare between heaven and earth. Hence, though some suffer from headache, some from stomachache, some from diabetes, some from anemia, and others from heart disease, gallstones, neuritis, or other ailments, yet all suffer for the same reason: simply because they have in one way or another moved away from their only fortress, the guidelines of Yahweh. This is the final diagnosis of all diseases. Stick close to Nature, and Nature will stick close to you.

I believe that most disease and death today is caused by disobedience to the Word of Yahweh. However, not all sickness and death is the result of individual sin. There are some things out of our control, such as environmental causes, accidents, and murder that can result in sickness and/or death. Beyond that, some people experience health challenges for no reason at all but to glorify the healing power of Yahweh through His Son Yeshua (John 9:1-3 and John 11:4). These things are beyond our control.

It is also important for me to point out that self-inflicted disease is not the same thing as pain and suffering. There can be much suffering and pain within disease; however, sometimes Yahweh puts those obedient to His guide through pain and suffering. These people understand their trials are for the glory of Yahweh and can enjoy peace during their discomfort. However, when someone is sick as a result of his sinful nature, he will never find peace during his trials.

It is easy to confuse disease with pain and suffering because they usually go together hand in hand. None of them were in Yahweh's original plan for man; however, because of Adam and Eve's disobedience to Yahweh, we were punished for their iniquity with pain and suffering in some areas of our lives as stated in Genesis 3:16-17, but we were never supposed to suffer with the massive amount of disease we experience today.

We are responsible for the choices we make. With the freedom of Yahweh comes responsibility. Our way of living has to be transformed. Our whole lives have to change not by our own efforts, but by Yahweh's. And along the way, we can realize that we can make the journey harder or easier by choosing to live lives that will produce disease or avoid disease.

As stated earlier, self-inflicted disease is not the same thing as pain and suffering. If our personal choices are not in line with the Scriptures, however, it can lead to all three (pain, suffering, and disease); but of the three, self-inflicted disease is the direct result of our own unrighteous action. If we listen and obey His guide, we would be free from the self-inflicted diseases of the world that so many people today suffer from, for we were wonderfully created in the image of Yahweh.

> *Thank You for making me so wonderfully complex! Your workmanship is marvelous — and how well I know it.* —Psalms 139:14 [NLT]

> *So Yahweh created humankind in His own image; in the image of Yahweh He created him: male and female He created them.* —Genesis 1:27

> *Yahweh saw everything that He had made, and indeed it was very good.* —Genesis 1:31

Disease and *wonderful* are opposites. Yahweh's image is good, sickness is not good. Disease as we know it today has gone far from Yahweh's original guide. Genesis 1:26 and 1:28 tell us that we humans we are to rule over every living organism. That is a command from Yahweh!

It was never Yahweh's plan for us to be overtaken by disease and disease organisms, but today that is what is happening. We are being destroyed, and we don't even realize it. Not only has it happened, it continues to happen so often that people accept it and consider it normal. It is not even odd any more. Viruses have gotten way out of control according to Yahweh's plan only because we have let them. If you accept the unnatural long enough, it starts to appear natural, but that's just the appearance. That is what has happened with the viruses and diseases that we suffer from today.

No matter how sick someone is, he can turn his health around if he gets back to the message of the Scriptures. It is a requirement of Yahweh that we possess the power built within us to overcome all germs and diseases. In Genesis 1:28, our Creator blessed humanity to be fruitful, to multiply, and to fill the earth. Genesis 1:28 also says we are to subdue and have dominion over every living thing. That includes cancer, bacteria, viruses, parasites, and other microorganisms that cause illness and disease.

Yahweh clearly tells how to avoid getting disease:

> *He said, "If you will listen intently to the voice of Yahweh your Creator, do what He considers right, pay attention to His commands and observe His laws, I will not afflict you with any of the diseases I brought on the Egyptians; because I am Yahweh your healer."*
> —Exodus 15:26

The people of Egypt during the time of Abraham were a group of people living against Yahweh's guide, and thus they suffered much disease. Because many of the Israelites would not let go of the sinful ways they learned while they were living with the Egyptians, they suffered many of the same illnesses.

No matter where we come from, we are assured by His Word that we need not get diseases that are so common among the world today. But many people choose to live against His guide and suffer. Many people cry out to Yahweh when they get sick and say, "Why me?" Disease is self-inflicted. The Scriptures tell us in many verses why we get sick. Here is one of the most obvious:

> Hear the word of Yahweh, O People of Israel! Yahweh has filed a lawsuit against you, saying: "There is no faithfulness, no kindness, and no knowledge of Elohim in your land.
>
> "You curse and lie and kill and steal and commit adultery. There is violence everywhere, with one murder after another.
>
> "That is why your land is not producing. It is filled with sadness, and all living things are becoming sick and dying. Even the animals, birds, and fish have begun to disappear." —Hosea 4:1-3 [NLT]

Now, we have Exodus 15:26 telling us what will happen if we do not follow Yahweh's guide, and we have Hosea 4:1-3 showing us clearly what is happening because we didn't listen to Exodus 15:26. In between Exodus and Hosea, we have many more great examples and warnings of where we went wrong.

Thanks to Yahweh's kindness, no matter how far off His path we have gotten, He gives us the instructions to get back in line with His Word.

Not all disease is due to rejection of Yahweh's Word; most is, but there are some people who are born with sicknesses for no other reason than to glorify Yahweh's Word. So if you are doing everything the Scriptures tell you to do and still suffering from an illness, take joy to know you may be one of the few chosen by Yahweh to glorify His mighty works, but please be careful not to mistake what I am saying here. *Most* people are not living His Word. Don't go by how you feel, saying you feel you are living the way He wants you to live. Even if you cannot confirm it with Scripture, most likely that's why you are sick!

I know some very righteous people who suffer with diseases. I've often asked myself, how could this be if they are so righteous? What I have realized with all these people, even though they have a disease, they have a certain peace about them because they know Yahweh, as opposed to people who flat out choose to live lives without Yahweh. When those people have disease, they have no peace or comfort.

> *Therefore, since the Messiah suffered physically, you too are to arm yourselves with the same attitude. For whoever has suffered physically is finished with sin.* —1 Peter 4:1

Sometimes the righteous are stricken with disease because Yahweh wants to keep them humble; however, people mostly get disease because in some area of their lives, they are not following Yahweh's instructions.

> *You will have to suffer only a little while; after that, Yahweh, who is full of grace, the one who called you to His eternal glory in union with the Messiah, will himself restore, establish and strengthen you and make you firm.* —1 Peter 5:10

If you do have a disease, I pray this book helps you with the information you need to get better. As a word of encouragement, we are to realize that all of Yahweh's faithful followers are assured of eternal life with Yeshua, where there will be no suffering (Revelation 21:4).

We need to realize it's Yahweh's will for us to be righteous and not only in our spiritual lives. John tells us it is Yahweh's will for us to be healthy physically as well as spiritually. The majority of people I know who are very righteous brothers have not followed, or are not following, the ideal food plan Yahweh laid out for us in the Torah.

> *Dear friend, I am praying that everything prosper with you and that you be in good health, as I know you are prospering spiritually.* —3 John 1:2

In treating disease, the first and most important thing is to find the root cause. Many people will almost always focus on the physical side of things first and try to improve their diets to some degree. Since they are most likely eating against the guidelines of Yahweh, they may show some improvement, but there are different root causes. If the root cause is emotional and you are trying to eat better to overcome your problem, you will not be successful. If you do suffer because of a low-quality diet, treating that issue spiritually will not get you the desired results. We must first identify the root cause. Is it physical, emotional, or spiritual?

I have found that in most people it is all three at the same time, so we must deal with all three. Remember, to overcome the blockage that is keeping us from experiencing Yahweh's blessing of good health and long life, we need to have knowledge and energy!

One of the common challenges I see people suffering from is struggling with the fact that they know they need to change their diets, but their flesh doesn't want to make the effort. Knowing you are eating a diet against Yahweh's ideal is not good enough. If you want to get rid of your illnesses, many times adjustments in your diet will help.

> *For a person who eats and drinks without recognizing the body eats and drinks judgment upon himself.*
>
> *This is why many among you are weak and sick, and some have died!* —1 Corinthians 11:29-30

Some people believe that since they know someone who lives an unrighteous life but does not experience sickness or disease, the message of this book can't be true. Yahweh loves us and has patience. Not everyone is going to get what he deserves right away. In fact, because of Yahweh's love for us, most people who are living lives against Yahweh's instructions have not experienced serious illness because Yahweh has not yet allowed the sickness they deserve to come upon them. But don't be deceived; this is because He loves us and wants to give us time to get our ways in order.

Sometimes I wonder if some people will never suffer the dreaded consequences — except for eternal death in consequence of their sin of disobedience, which in this life they seemed to have gotten away with. It's like a person who has lost pain sensation. It might seem good to not feel pain, but pain helps to alert us to a problem. Some don't feel pain as a result of what they are doing that may well lead to their deaths; whereas, if they did feel pain, they could have nipped the problem in the bud before it did them in.

CHAPTER 22

Healing according to the Scriptures: The Fear of Yahweh Leads to Life!

Yahweh my Creator, I cried out to You, and You provided healing for me. —Psalms 30:2

Once we make a covenant with Yahweh and stick to it, our past sins are wiped away and many times so are our sicknesses. There are many sick people today who accept Yeshua with their lips, but they go back on their word. They don't have the instructions of Yahweh on their hearts, and they continue to suffer.

As stated earlier, Yahweh wants us healthy; disease is not what He wanted for us. If you have children, you know that no matter how disobedient your children might have been in the past and no matter how much they suffer for it, never are you happy about their suffering. You will do anything possible to take away their pain, to help them avoid suffering more.

We are children of Yahweh, and in His love for us and His mercy, He gives us time to get our acts together. His gave us His Word to guide us. He gave us Yeshua to heal us. The name *Yeshua* means 'Yahweh's salvation'!

Why are we sick, and how can we be healed? This is all clearly stated in Psalms 107:17-20 and many other scriptures. The problem we have is that we are so occupied with the things of the world that we miss the words of Yahweh.

Having no time to study and pray and too lazy to obey, we are on a crash course for destruction. We are told in 1 John 2:15 not to love the ways of the world; if we do, Yahweh is not truly in us.

But as stated in Romans 8:11, if the Set-apart Spirit can make a dead man live, then it can certainly make a sick man well again!

There were foolish people who suffered affliction because of their crimes and sins;

> *they couldn't stand to eat anything; they were near the gates of death.*
>
> *In their trouble they cried to Yahweh, and He rescued them from their distress;*
>
> *He sent His Word and healed them, He delivered them from destruction.* —Psalms 107:17-20

Yeshua Heals

> *Yeshua went about all the towns and villages, teaching in their synagogues, proclaiming the Good News of the Kingdom, and healing every kind of disease and weakness.* —Matthew 9:35

<u>Yahweh</u>
Saves — from Sin
Heals — from Sickness
Delivers — from Satan

<u>Yeshua</u>
Teaches — knowledge that will save us
Preaches — the good news to heal us
Heals — by His redeeming blood

Use Yahweh's medicine and don't doubt in Yahweh! Many people today go to doctors first and use prayer as a last resort. We should not neglect Yahweh in favor of medical treatment. Yahweh creates the means of healing, both natural and supernatural, and wants us to keep Him as the focus of all healings. We see this example with Asa who went to physicians for healing but not to Yahweh.

> *In the thirty-ninth year of his reign, Asa suffered from a disease in his legs. It was a very serious disease, yet even with this disease he did not seek out Yahweh but turned to the physicians.* —2 Chronicles 16:12

The Result?

> *Asa slept with his ancestors, dying in the forty-first year of his reign.* —2 Chronicles 16:13

Asa is a good example of the person today who confesses with his lips that he accepts Yeshua as the Messiah. The new-found faith is well seen at first, but only the person who accepts Yeshua with the heart will persevere!

Asa was like the new believer today who lives a righteous life while it seems simple and easy, thinking there will be no trials, but a little study of the Word and time in the faith reveal that the righteous will be persecuted and shunned by the world. This revelation to the new believer, along with the distractions of the world and the deceptions of Satan, eventually gets people off track. Eventually many people who professed Yeshua as the Messiah end up choosing the easy way rather than the right way. As Shaul (Paul) said, many are called, but only few choose.

Asa obeyed Yahweh during the first ten years of his reign. He carried out a partially successful effort to abolish idolatry and deposed his idolatrous grandmother, Maacah. All seemed to be going well. In Asa's greatest act of faithfulness in battle against the Ethiopians, the odds seemed impossible for Asa to win. Asa recognized his need to depend on Yahweh, and he prayed to Yahweh! That was the high point of Asa's life, but things went sour from there. Asa made alliances with foreign nations and evil people and responded with rage when confronted about his sin.

It is one thing to profess Yeshua as our Messiah and to live a righteous life for a certain time, but it's consistency that counts. Who is in it for the long run? Sick people are weak. Unfaithful, unwise, and disobedient people are weaker. A healthy person is a strong person.

> *And if the Spirit of the One who raised Yeshua from the dead is living in you, then the One who raised the Messiah Yeshua from the dead will also give life to your mortal bodies through His Spirit living in you.* —Romans 8:11

Earlier in this book, I said many times in the Scriptures you can replace the word 'evil' with the word 'sickness', and it would fit nicely in those places. Well, for 'health' we can use the word 'strength', and it would fit nicely in many places as well. Also, if strength is health, then 'weakness' can mean 'sickness'. We can first see an example of this in Judges with Samson.

Finally, Samson shared his secret with her. "My hair has never been cut," he confessed, "for I was dedicated to Yahweh as a Nazarite from birth. If my head were shaved, my strength [health] would leave me, and I would become as weak [sick] as anyone else" (Judges 16:17).

> *A wise man is strong* [healthy]; *yes, a man of knowledge grows in strength* [health]. —Proverbs 24:5
>
> *Yahweh is my strength* [health] *and protection; He makes my way go straight.* —2 Samuel 22:33

An important key to healing is to experience the peace, the shalom, of Yahweh. The opposite of this peace is to be at war.

> *Yahweh gives strength* [health] *to His people; Yahweh blesses His people with peace.* —Psalms 29:11 [NIV]

Now let's take one last look at Asa's life and how all this relates.

> *For the eyes of Yahweh move here and there throughout the whole earth, to show himself strong* [healing] *on behalf of those who are wholehearted toward Him. You acted foolishly in this regard; for from now on, you will have war."* —2 Chronicles 16:9

War is the opposite of peace. The verse says Yahweh looks to strengthen, or heal, those whose hearts are fully committed to him. What is the result of people who are not fully committed?

> *He has broken my strength* [health] *in mid-course, He has cut short my days.* —Psalms 102:23

So we need Yahweh's strength to heal! We need to be made stronger, not weaker, as we are weaker in sickness and stronger in health.

Faith, knowledge, wisdom, understanding, obedience, and consistency are all important keys to health, but what exactly did Yahweh give us to help heal us if we are already sick? What was Yahweh's prescribed medicine for our healing?

Yahweh's Medicine
Herbs, Oils, and Prayer

We have already covered the topic of herbs, the greens that are so healing to the body. There is another important verse that mentions the healing of green leaves.

> *Between the main street and the river was the Tree of Life producing twelve kinds of fruit, a different kind every month; and the leaves of the tree were for healing the nations.* —Revelation 22:2

One of the final things we are told in the Scriptures is that the leaves of the tree are used for the healing of all. There are many different ideas about what this means, but even if Yahweh was using this as a metaphor, He did so most likely because it is clear that green herbs, leaves, and grass are healing for our bodies.

Ezekiel provides us with information to confirm this, and there are many other scriptures that talk about the importance of green leaves as our medicine.

> *On both riverbanks will grow all kinds of trees for food; their leaves will not dry up, nor will their fruit fail. There will be a different kind of fruit each month, because the water flows from the sanctuary, so that this fruit will be edible, and the leaves will have healing properties.* —Ezekiel 47:12

Amongst all the foods that are best for our bodies, I let everyone know about the great healing herbs that are available to us. I would usually send someone to an herb shop before the doctor. The greatest herb shops can be found right in our own neighborhoods. There are wild weeds and green herbs that are all over empty lots and back yards that people have no idea about. A good study of wild edible herbs will surprise most people about how many great edible herbs are around them that they can simply pick and put into a salad. Of course there are herb shops where you can buy certain herbs for medicine if we need them. The bottom line is herbs should be our first line of defense in our healing or in just staying well.

Now let's look at a verse that has in it the healing power of oil and prayer.

> *Is someone among you in trouble? He should pray. Is someone feeling good? He should sing songs of praise.*

> *Is someone among you ill? He should call for the elders of the congregation. They will pray for him and rub olive oil on him in the name of the Creator.*
>
> *The prayer offered with trust will heal the one who is ill — the Creator will restore his health; and if he has committed sins, he will be forgiven.*
>
> *Therefore, openly acknowledge your sins to one another, and pray for each other, so that you may be healed. The prayer of a righteous person is powerful and effective.* —James 5:13-16

The Healing Power of Anointing Oils

In the Scriptures, anointing oils were used as both a medicine (Luke 10:34) and a symbol of the spirit of Yahweh. (As used in anointing kings, see 1 Samuel 16:1-13.) This oil can represent both the medical and the spiritual spheres of life. Believers should not separate the physical and the spiritual. Yeshua is Elohim over both the body and the spirit.

In the Talmud, olive oil symbolizes knowledge of the Torah, which provides spiritual illumination. Oil is also the symbol of joy (in Psalms 45:7), so it is called the "oil of gladness."

Oil is a picture of the Set-apart Spirit. By anointing with oil, the elders are claiming Yahweh's promises that the Set-apart Spirit will minister to the health and life of the sick child of Yahweh.

Today, science is catching up to Yahweh's Scriptures that reveal to us what we need to stay healthy and to heal us if we are sick. The food mentioned in the Scriptures as best for man is now being confirmed by science. As man today spends millions of dollars looking for a magic medicine to heal our sicknesses, Yahweh's great wisdom reveals the oils mentioned in the Scriptures were antiviral, antibacterial, antifungal, anti-infectious, anti-inflammatory, antiseptic, antimicrobial, antineuralgic, antirheumatic, and immune stimulating. Herbs and oils are Yahweh's healing medicine. If used correctly, they have no harmful side effects and are more cost effective than man's medicine. Viruses do not become resistant to oils as they do to modern-day synthetic antibiotic drugs.

There are numerous references to essential oils (or the plants they are derived from) in the Scriptures. Some precious oils, such as frankincense, myrrh, galbanum, rosemary, hyssop, cassia, cinnamon, and spikenard were used for anointing and healing of the sick.

> *Is there no medicine in Gilead? Is there no physician there?*
> —Jeremiah 8:22 [NLT]

Recent excavation of the ancient city Gilead has unearthed the remains of a fortresslike building used for the manufacture of balsam oil. This "balm of Gilead" noted in Jeremiah 8:22 had long been famous in antiquity for its nearly miraculous properties to *heal wounds*. In fact, the balsam oil of Gilead was so famous that the conquering Roman emperor Titus (79-81 A.D.), after conquering Gilead, displayed branches from Gilead's balsam trees in his triumphal march through Rome.

The anointing oils of the Scriptures are known today as essential oils. In the Scriptures, they are also referred to as "fragrances," "odors," "ointments," "aromas," "perfumes," or "sweet savors." At least 33 different essential oils or aromatic oil-producing plants are mentioned, along with over 600 references in the Scriptures to oils and/or the aromatic plants from which they were extracted. I have personally used an array of essential oils and experienced healing. I have also seen others who have used them to their benefit as well. There is enough proof out there to confirm that the healing oils of the Scriptures are Yahweh's medicine.

The Healing Power of Prayer and Faith

Heal me, Yahweh, and I will be healed; save me, and I will be saved, for You are my praise. —Jeremiah 17:14

If Yahweh is our Doctor and His Word, or salvation (Yeshua), the medicine, prayer would be the key that opens up the doctor's office. Our part of the covenant we made with Yahweh was to please Him, and nothing pleases Him more than us coming to him in prayer with humble hearts. Regardless of our struggles, our trials, or our shortcomings, Yahweh delights when we seek

Him to help us. When we acknowledge Him first and foremost, He will reward our loving hearts.

> *Yahweh detests the sacrifices of the wicked but delights in the prayers of the upright.* —Proverbs 15:8
>
> *Yahweh is far from the wicked, but He listens to the prayer of the righteous.* —Proverbs 15:29
>
> *Yahweh is close to all who call on Him, to all who sincerely call on Him.*
> *He fulfills the desire of those who fear Him; He hears their cry and saves them.*
> *Yahweh protects all who love Him, but all the wicked He destroys.*
> —Psalms 145:18-20

As we can see, Yahweh loves it when we pray to Him, and He hears us and grants us our desires. If our hearts are righteous, we will be led to ask for only what is good in Yahweh's sight. Yahweh rejects the prayers of the unrighteous because of their selfish prayers. Yahweh rescues and protects the righteous who call to Him. The key is communication. We must communicate with Yahweh.

He doesn't need to hear our needs; He knows exactly what we need. He doesn't need to hear our thoughts; He knows exactly what we are thinking. He doesn't need us for anything. When we realize what Yahweh has done and continues to do for us every day, when we rejoice in His love for us and come to Him and thank Him day and night, then Yahweh rejoices in us and will heal us!

> *Don't worry about anything; on the contrary, make your requests known to Yahweh by prayer and petition, with thanksgiving.*
>
> *Then Yahweh's shalom, passing all understanding, will keep your hearts and minds safe in union with the Messiah Yeshua.*
> —Philippians 4:6-7

Shalom, peace, is health! Replace worry with prayer and enjoy Yahweh's shalom!

Keep persisting in prayer, staying alert in it and being thankful.
—Colossians 4:2

This is the confidence we have in His presence: if we ask anything that accords with His will, He hears us.
And if we know that He hears us — whatever we ask — then we know that we have what we have asked from Him. —1 John 5:14-15

When it comes to healing and the Scriptures, Yahweh gives us the healthy food to eat, the healing herbs to consume, and the anointing oils to use, but when we pray, we are giving back to Yahweh. That's when we will experience complete healing! Hallelu-Yah!

Ways to Treat Disease: Doctor or Yahweh

There are two ways to treat disease: by going to the doctor or by seeking Yahweh. First we'll look at the world's way, going to the doctor.

The World's Way: Going to the Doctor

The First Commandment is, "Have no other elohim before Me." When we hold a doctor in such high esteem, it's doing just that. People today break this Commandment when they run to the doctor when they get sick and pray to Yahweh only after everything the doctor tells them to do is not working. We need to go to Yahweh first and seek His will for us. Going to the doctor when you are sick is like taking your car to the dentist when it breaks down. We need to use the guide in the glove compartment to get well again.

People today have become unfaithful in Yahweh and have decided to make their doctors their idols. Whatever doctors say is taken as the best answer. Most doctors know very little about health and healing. Their training in medical school concerns diseases and medicine. In fact, some of the unhealthiest places in the world are hospitals. Most doctors are trained to control disease, not heal it.

Now I'm not saying all doctors are bad. When considering

emergency doctors and other special cases, such as spinal cord injuries, may Yahweh bless them. But if I'm going to get sick due to my own self-indulgence, a drug prescribed by a doctor is not a healthful cure. Yahweh's cure is quite the opposite. "Let thy food be thy medicine, and medicine be thy food," Hippocrates said.

Yahweh made our bodies to heal from all disease by resting and eating only healthful foods. Doctors keep us very busy consuming some of the worst stuff ever invented.

> *Among them was a woman who had had a hemorrhage for twelve years*
>
> *and had suffered a great deal under many physicians. She had spent her life savings; yet instead of improving, she had grown worse.* —Mark 5:25-26

The Way of Yahweh

The other way to treat disease is seeking Yahweh. Listen to His Spirit that dwells within you. You know you're listening to the right Spirit because there is no confusion or doubt in His healing power.

> *Abraham prayed to Yahweh, and Yahweh healed.* —Genesis 20:17
>
> *I am Yahweh your healer.* —Exodus 15:26
>
> *He forgives all your offenses, He heals all your diseases.* —Psalms 103:3

There is no better doctor than Yahweh and no better medicine than prayer and the Word of Yahweh.

> *He preserves our lives and keeps our feet from stumbling.* —Psalms 66:9

Yahweh sent His Son to heal all our diseases if we accept the healing.

> *Yeshua went all over the Galilee teaching in their synagogues, proclaiming the Good News of the Kingdom, and healing people from every kind of disease and sickness.* —Matthew 4:23

What doctor do you know that can heal every kind of disease?

It is better to trust in Yahweh than to put confidence in man.
—Psalms 118:8 [NKJV]

The Medicine of Yahweh

People today listen to a doctor's exact words even if they don't make sense to them. If a doctor tells people to take medicine in the middle of the night, they will set their alarm clocks just to make sure they do it correctly. If the doctor tells them they must take food with their drugs, people will eat even if they are not hungry, and so on.

Why listen to a doctor? The prescription usually causes more problems than it cures. We need to listen and obey our Creator to be healthy!

Yahweh our Father and Creator of everything in the world has given us the greatest prescription for good health in His book of wisdom (Proverbs). This is not a book we should just glance over quickly. Careful attention should be given when reading these next verses. I do believe that if people listened and followed the instructions in these next verses as well as they listen to and follow the advice of some strange doctor, sickness and disease would almost disappear off the face of this earth.

> *My son, give attention to My words; incline your ear to My sayings.*
>
> *Do not let them depart from your eyes; keep them in the midst of your heart.*
>
> *For they are life to those who find them, and health to all their flesh.*
> —Proverbs 4:20-22 [NKJV]

This is the formula, or medicine, we need to overcome all our illnesses and discomforts.

• My son, listen to My Words: Yahweh is telling us, even commanding us, to listen to, or to hear, what He is saying. Deuteronomy 28:15 says, "If you will not listen to Yahweh and do His commands ... curses shall come upon you."

What more needs to be said? The answer is right there. Sickness is a curse, and we now have the information to cure it. But listening alone won't do it. There is more to the cure.

• Incline your ear to My sayings: Here Yahweh is telling us not just to hear what He's saying, but to pay attention to what is being said, to stay focused on His Word and not get sidetracked. We must also incline (bend) our ways to His sayings so we can understand. Not only our ways but our hearts!

> *Incline my heart to Your testimonies, and not to covetousness.*
> —Psalms 119:36 [NKJV]

• Let them not depart from your eyes: When man first sinned, his eyes became open to all the sins of the world. The temptations of this world can get us very sick if we give in to them. Here Yahweh is telling us to stay focused on His laws, His commandments, and not to look elsewhere.

> *Turn my eyes away from worthless things; with Your ways, give me life.* —Psalms 119:37

People's attentions today have strayed very far from focusing on Yahweh. What people watch, how they dress, and whom they associate with go completely against Yahweh's instructions. Condoning worldly behavior, partaking in man-made traditions, and idolizing pagan gods have become the norm! We take prayer out of our schools and courts, replace faith with magic, and accept pagan practices while rejecting the way of our Creator, and still we wonder why we suffer?

We have replaced a moral system that assures us the highest-quality health with an immoral system that leads to destruction. Where have we learned this behavior? Why have we let this happen, and why don't we do anything to stop it? We blame our disobedient lifestyles on addiction, excuse it with grace, and live in ignorance of what is really going on. It's time for a reality check! What are we filling our minds with? The answer can reveal how so many self-professed Christians are so easily led astray today.

- Guard them in the midst of your heart: I feel this is one of the most important of all the scriptures concerning our health. This is also what most people are missing and the reason so many people in the churches and assemblies are sick and diseased. The word 'guard' is so powerful here. It confirms all the scriptures. To guard means to 'defend'. We are to defend His Word always. It is good to do His Word, but we can't stop there.

If anyone were to spread false gossip about your children or make up ugly rumors about your spouse, chances are you wouldn't take it lightly. You would speak up and say something. Well, this is what we are told to do in Proverbs 4:23.

There are many ways to guard His Word. One of the best ways I have found to do so is to teach the Word. Whenever we teach the Word, we are guarding it. It's when we say nothing that we are not following the Word. In Romans 2:13, it is written, "For it is not merely knowing the law that brings Yahweh's approval. Those who obey the law will be declared right in Yahweh's sight."

We need to wake up and do like Shaul (Paul) did in Acts 13:9-10 when he was in the presence of a sorcerer named Elymas. He looked him right in the eye and said, "You son of the devil, full of every sort of deceit and fraud, and enemy of all that is good! Will you never stop perverting the true ways of Yahweh?"

We may not have the opportunity to look everyone in the eye, but we can set an example by the message we preach and by our actions that back it up. There are times we can approach a person in a kindly way, but do not be afraid of offending him. Just pray to Yahweh to show you what approach to take, and let Him give you the courage to do so.

- For they are life to those who find them: Many people today are lost and searching, but the answer is in His Word. Those who find it will find a spiritual life like never before!

For he who finds Me finds life and obtains the favor of Yahweh.
But he who misses Me harms himself; all who hate Me love death."
—Proverbs 8:35-36

- And healing to all their flesh: The discipline of Yahweh is healing to all our flesh. We are punished and suffer for our sins;

but if we are wise, we learn from that punishment. We don't continue to commit the same sins. Our physical punishment cleanses away evil. Yahweh's discipline purifies our hearts.

> *Blows that wound purge away evil, yes, beatings* [cleanse] *one's inmost being.* —Proverbs 20:30

> *He restores my inner person. He guides me in right paths for the sake of His own name.*
> *Even if I pass through death-dark ravines, I will fear no disaster; for You are with me; Your rod and staff reassure me.* —Psalms 23:3-4

Not just healing for some of your sicknesses, He will heal *all* your flesh!

Go to Yahweh and seek His will always, before running to the doctor to heal your illness. Running to the doctor is just another crazy custom of this world. Run to Yahweh! He will give you wisdom and healing to all your flesh.

Cleansing your Temple

Hopefully by now you will realize that you don't need to consume much food if you plan your diet with wisdom. However, what is factual and practical is not always the same thing. I have a hard time convincing people about the health benefits of eating less food less often, but even the people I do convince still see no way to do it. They just can't seem to break the addiction that has been with them for so long.

The good news is that unless you are very sick, you don't have to make the change overnight. Making the needed changes gradually over time can help anyone easily make the necessary adjustments without even realizing what he has done. For example, if you give up just one harmful food a month, you will have given up over one year twelve harmful foods that you were used to consuming. If you gave up those twelve foods overnight at the same time, it would have been a much bigger challenge.

In this part of the book, I want to share with you some tips on how to gradually reduce the amount of food you consume without making such a drastic, quick change. You first have to get the thinking out of your mind of what people teach about more being better. That's not always the case. In the case of nutrition, your body can use only so much, and everything else is going to be stored as fat or go to waste. A healthy, clean body requires only small amounts of nutriment to keep things in great working order.

However, a toxic body requires more food sometimes, not because it needs more nutrients, but because the extra food may slow down the detoxification to where it is not too uncomfortable for the person. It's a cycle that goes round and round because the ideal way a person can detox is to consume less. It all comes down to adjustments. It has taken you a very long time to get to the point where you can consume as much food you do as often as you do, so it will take some time to reverse and become used to consuming less. It's not only physical; we also need to consider the social and emotional changes that will adjust during this process.

Clean your temple inside and out.
Detoxifying

Cleaning your body internally requires it to go through a detoxification. You might look worse before you look better, and you'll feel worse before you feel better while your body is undergoing detoxification. This scares many people, but only because they don't understand detoxification. Many worry about detoxification, thinking it's a bad sign, but it's a good sign.

You'll understand detoxification if you remember this: "Energy is always noted in its expenditure, never in its accumulation. Whenever one feels stronger, he is often getting weaker, because he is expending his strength more rapidly. On the contrary, when feeling weakest, strength is often accumulating most rapidly. It is accumulating and hence unnoticed."

That piece of information can help so many people understand why eating healthfully and cleaning out will sometimes make them feel worse before they feel better. Healing requires consuming the foods that are best for your body. The best way to avoid bodily dehydration is to eat the foods that will keep your body clean and free of excess mucus and slime.

The more water you have in your body, the cleaner you will be. If water is your soap, then you want to drink a lot of it to stay clean and free of debris. The best foods for the human body are those that contain the most water (liquid). Water will help you stay clean and remove the dirt that has been there for so long causing disease and discomfort.

CHAPTER 23

The Formula for Health: He Will Heal All Diseases

My people are destroyed for lack of knowledge. —Hosea 4:6 [NKJV]

People today are used to overeating. They are addicted to the taste, flavors, and consistency of food, and it often seems it's the only way to put a smile on someone's face until finished, often with a food hangover.

Besides the physical addictions, there is something else that is convincing people to eat more than they need. That is lack of knowledge. It is important to understand Yahweh's schedule and believe it is best for everyone, not just for a few chosen people. When people have a hard time giving up their pleasures, they often make excuses to keep indulging them. Concerning food, people will say they need more and more and more. You get the point.

When people see I suggest only two meals a day, many ask me about how they will get energy if they don't eat so much. We don't get as much energy from food as we think. In fact, it takes more energy for the body to digest food many times than what we are getting from it. The reason we often feel a burst of energy after eating is that food stimulates us. No matter what we eat, we get stimulation from food; but if we consume food with stimulants in it, the temporary effect is even more unbalancing.

This stimulation may seem good, but what price are we paying? After much thinking and prayer about what is going on today with health, I see many people addicted to stimulating ingredients in food, such as sugar and caffeine. All these habits usually lead to two major problems: blood sugar issues and adrenal exhaustion. It is a never-ending cycle because this all leads up to a major stress on the rest of the body. But then on the same hand, it is the stress that leads to overeating.

To be healthy, we need to support the immune system of the body and not add stress to it. Once we overstress our nervous systems, we start burning nutrients in excess. This will lead to deficiencies, depression, and yes, insomnia. Now the door will be open to many other issues.

As a result of eating more often than we need to and on a different timetable than Yahweh advises, the common result of overeating and eating too late at night is lack of rest and sleep. This will usually result in some form of adrenal fatigue. Adrenal fatigue is the most common, but misidentified, illness today.

I've been on a good quality diet for many years. I felt good but should have felt better. It wasn't until I broke the addiction to my late night eating that I started to feel better. I was happy with the new results, but I was also interested to understand why. I wanted to know beyond the fact that I was able to sleep better why I felt so much better. One of the reasons I wanted to figure this out was also to help others overcome health challenges as well.

It had been my understanding that energy was another word for health, based on research for my book *The Formula for Health*. I am clear to warn everyone that energy and stimulation are two different things. Energy is the result we get when we eat a good diet, get the proper amount of rest, and live a healthy lifestyle. Simulation is the result of needing to take or do something to make us feel a spark of energy, but it's a false sense of energy in a way. I have found most people are not doing too well in the energy field and were relying more and more on stimulants to keep them feeling good.

To help you understand about food and health, I would like to briefly introduce you to my formula for health. This is just an overview, but it should supply you with some understanding of how the body works. If you would like to study the subject more, you can read my book *Paul Nison's Raw Food Formula for Health*.

There is a health formula that conveys the health principles found in the Scriptures. Understanding this health formula will help you comprehend how the body stays healthy and what foods are best to consume. Here it is:

Power − Obstruction = Vitality

Another way to say it would be:

Health − Disease = Wellness

Here is how the formula works. *Power* is 'health', or as I prefer to refer to it, 'energy'. I don't mean energy as in stimulation, but rather the energy you get when you've had the proper sleep and nutrition. *Obstruction* is 'any stress or dis-ease of the body'. And *Vitality* is 'wellness', or the level of health we experience. So:

Health − Disease = Wellness

In other words, your degree of wellness, or vitality, is what's left of your health when you "subtract" any sickness or discomfort. For example, if you're a very healthy person, but happen to get a cold, you still have a good supply of overall wellness. But if you don't eat right, don't sleep enough, and then get a cold, you'll have less vitality and ability to heal. Obviously, the healthier you are, the more vitality you will have to help you when you get sick.

As long as the body is able to maintain enough power/health to remove the obstruction/disease, there is going to be some degree of vitality/wellness. If the obstruction/disease becomes greater than your power/health, you won't have the energy to get rid of the obstruction.

The greater the obstruction, the more likely the disease will reach an advanced stage. So the state of our health is determined by the degree of this vital energy we have left after the body has used its power to get rid of the waste. If the body runs out of energy to supply the power, waste will build up more quickly. Because the body no longer has enough energy to eliminate the buildup of toxic substances, an excess amount of toxins accumulates in the blood. Soon, we're experiencing the first stages of disease.

If Power − Obstruction = Vitality, or the amount of health we have is equal to Power - Obstruction, too little power and too much obstruction will put us into very diseased states.

This formula is so important to understand because the most common obstruction we have is what we put into our bodies. The food we consume, the type, the amount, and its timing all contribute to the obstruction. Simply, good health is living with the least amount of obstruction.

The only obstruction-free diet is the divine diet mapped out by our wonderful Maker, Yahweh. His nutrition plan consists of only the highest-quality foods, while showing us the ideal times to consume them to conserve the most energy possible. Remember, as long as we have energy to get rid of any obstructions, we will be in a state of health.

The key to health from a physical standpoint is taking in as many nutrients as necessary while using as little power as possible to digest them, and also keeping the body's internal environment as clean as possible. A diet found in Genesis 1:29, raw fruits and vegetables, does just that.

Fruits and vegetables require the least amount of the body's energy, yet they provide the most nutrients. In other words, you get more bang for your digestive buck with fruits and vegetables than with any other foods. They are your best source of energy.

PART 6

In the End It Will Be As It Was at the Beginning

At the beginning I announce the end, proclaim in advance things not yet done; and I say that My plan will hold, I will do everything I please to do. —Isaiah 46:10

"Declaring the end out of the beginning and out of ancient times."

CHAPTER 24

Putting a Plan Together:
Seek the Kingdom of Yahweh above All Things!

For Yahweh watches over the way of the righteous. —Psalms 1:6

Diet and the Scriptures

Hopefully after getting the knowledge in this book about what the Scriptures have to say about diet, you now understand that eating large amounts of food and/or highly processed and fortified foods is not what Yahweh wants. They will cause the body to work very hard to get what it needs. When a sufficient quantity of Yahweh's high-quality natural foods is consumed, the body gets what it needs, and only very small amounts are needed.

What it really comes down to is that we were made with a wonderful, built-in intelligence. The body doesn't know the names or forms of foods you're eating. It simply takes what it needs and gets rid of the rest. Let's eat foods that have an abundance of goodness the body can use and as little as possible that will go to waste.

A wise tip when changing your diet would be to go at your own pace. Make changes when you feel you're ready physically and mentally. Otherwise, you'll run into some problems. No two people are in the same place at the same time. You must move at your own pace, not at someone else's. If you go too slowly, you won't see the results. If you go too fast, you won't enjoy the changes.

A Very Good Tip to Help You Get Started

Decide on set mealtimes each day, and plan your meals ahead of time. Years ago, I used to suggest people eat only when hungry. This failed because people overate so much that if they missed one meal, they felt hungry. However, this was not true hunger but habit hunger. We could go for weeks without any food before feeling true hunger, but people are so used to eating so many meals that if they miss only one, they don't know how to react. Slowly but surely, cut back on the number of meals you eat, consume only the highest-quality food, and your health will improve.

Remember: Health doesn't begin with what we add to our diets, but with what we leave out. If we take care of our bodies, if we consistently avoid putting things into them that don't belong, we will become clean and healthy.

The surest way to know whether or not a food belongs in the body is to listen to your body when it's still in its clean stages, or when it returns to cleanliness.

Most people today have no idea what true health is, because everyone around them is also sick. Since sickness looks so normal, they accept it and think that's what health is. I invite you to try each diet plan of Yahweh and then try man's diet plans. See for yourself which way you feel best.

If you have come to any conclusion about the views already, and if you have any pain or disease in your life from a physical standpoint, I encourage you to realize that may not be Yahweh's perfect will for you. And if you are eating the way you feel Yahweh wants you to and feel wonderful about it physically, emotionally, and spiritually, that's great; but don't mistake health for what we see today.

People look at stimulation as energy, take drugs as cures, and overeat to suppress their pain. That is not the health I'm talking about. The Scriptures are quite clear about what is the best way to eat, what way is accepted but not ideal, and what way is completely against Yahweh's Torah. I pray we all get right with the Word so we can receive His true and full blessing.

> *And when the wicked person turns away from all the wickedness he has committed and does what is lawful and right, he will save his life.*
>
> *Because he thinks it over and repents of all the transgressions he committed, he will certainly live, not die.* —Ezekiel 18:27-28

Now that we have all this information along with Yahweh's Torah as our guide, what do we do next? We need a plan to follow to make our transition to healthier lives successful. These next pages will be that plan. This plan is suggested, but adjustments for each person can be made based on physical limitations, work schedule, and other factors. These suggestions are just a model for each person to build his own plan.

For example, a person with children will not have as much time and freedom as a single person. Or a person working a night job cannot go to sleep at the same time as a person with a day job. The suggestions in this plan are the most ideal, based on Yahweh's Torah; so do your best to stick as closely as possible to them, but don't completely avoid them if you cannot follow them 100%.

Your Daily Diet: Cleansing, Transition, and Maintenance

The best way to make a simple and easy transition to a better quality diet is to be consistent, continue to gain knowledge, and enjoy experiencing all the new foods and tastes. Once you clean your body of many of the toxins you've put into it during years past, you can go on a maintenance diet. But before you go on a maintenance diet, you have to know where you are, where you want to be, and how you will get there. You need a plan. There are three stages to success: cleansing, transition, and maintenance. Following are suggestions for each of these three phases.

The Cleansing Diet (One Day to Three Months)

Technically, the Transitional Diet and the Cleansing Diet can be considered as one and the same, in that both cleanse the system. Do not rush into things you're not sure of. There is no need to exceed your understanding of cleansing. As long as you go at a good pace, you should avoid any possible issues that may come up with cleansing too fast.

The Cleansing Diet period can encompass any or all of the following: fasting, juicing, blending, and limiting sugar. There are many other practices that can be done in addition to these food recommendations, such as herbal cleanses, enemas, colonics, and other cleansing treatments, but for the purposes of this book, I'm focusing only on the food aspects. I suggest reading further on those other topics. Adding the nonfood treatments to my recommended cleansing diet will enhance any cleanse and give you the best results.

You can go on a cleansing diet any time. Whenever you feel the need over the years, you can always return to do a shorter or longer cleanse. During a cleansing diet, eat as simply as possible, leaving out heavy and miscombined foods, limiting your sugar intake, and avoiding all meat, eggs, and dairy products during the cleansing stage.

The quickest way to cleanse is not to eat at all. This is called a fast. I've met individuals who regularly fast for a few days all the way up to a few weeks. A three-day fast is recommended during the cleansing stages. The best suggestion for a cleanse and a maintenance diet is to fast one whole day each week.

Fasting could mean abstaining from solid food and just juicing, or doing a complete fast and abstaining from all food. Eating no food or beverages and just having water would be the most cleansing, but the detoxification process can produce more acute symptoms that are unpleasant to experience. Unless one can relax and stay in bed for three days, I recommend a juice diet, only consuming green vegetable juices for three days. Fruit juices are too high in sugar, so I prefer green vegetable juices.

The Transitional Diet (One to Two Years)

While going along on a Transitional Diet at a good pace, your body will slowly cleanse. The less you eat, the more quickly your body will clean itself out. Once you've eliminated harmful foods, your body will become stronger than when you started. This is an excellent time to begin an even more cleansing diet.

At this stage, you will rid yourself of the toxins that have built up in your system. It is a wise idea to continue eating only healthful foods once you clean out so that the toxins you rid your body of don't return. Once your body is cleansed, you can move to more of a maintenance diet. It is important to clean out before trying to rebuild.

For the transitional stage, just about any raw and organic fruit or vegetable is fine. At this stage, if animals or animal products are consumed, I suggest limiting them. As you get healthier, you'll eventually want to refine your diet, focusing not only on the quality of your food, but also on its quantity.

It would also be worthwhile to heed the principles of food combining, limiting the amount of fat and sugar and focusing on more leafy green vegetables. (If you're faced with a specific health challenge, you may have to go to the next stage sooner; if not, you can enjoy this stage as long as you have to, but do your best not to go beyond two years in this stage).

During a Transitional Diet, slight symptoms of discomfort may appear as part of the process. Those who don't understand how the body works might take these symptoms as negative signs. This is one reason it's so vital to understand the relationship between health and nutrition before getting ahead of oneself. That is the biggest common mistake made by those on a Transitional Diet and the reason many "give up."

These symptoms are magnified to an even greater extent on a Cleansing Diet. You should not attempt a Cleansing Diet until you've understood what these symptoms mean. If a Transitional Diet is done at a moderate pace, then no danger should be encountered. If one goes too fast, there is always some challenge, but there are even more challenges during the Cleansing Diet.

The Maintenance Diet (for Life)

You want to get to a point where you are following this stage more often than the other stages. Make sure you've cleansed and detoxified before going to this stage. It's an individually tailored diet geared to your lifestyle. This stage should be different from the Transitional and the Cleansing Diets. It should consist of foods from the best sources available, hopefully food that is organic and fresh. Do the best you can! As the years go by, you'll naturally want to simplify your diet more and more.

The key when it comes to diet is keeping the body supplied with the nutrients it needs while conserving as much energy as possible.

I suggest eating only two meals a day with no snacking between meals and not eating when dark outside. If you're accustomed to three meals a day, this may take some getting used to; but once high-quality food is consumed with the body cleaned out, you'll find that a meal's worth of food is enough. You should not have a desire for food at other times of the day. If you feel this is too much of a change and need three meals a day, just make sure your last meal is eaten by 7 p.m. Do *not* consume food after 7 p.m. Of course, you don't have to be completely rigid about this — sometimes it cannot be helped — but as a general rule, try not to eat too late.

Also, do not drink water *with* your meals. Drink one hour before or one hour after your meals, but not with your meals. Try to get at least eight hours of sleep a night.

On the following page is a daily journal to keep track of how the changes are going and any issues or challenges that might arise. Writing down the information will help keep you on track. I suggest making a copy of the journal and each day filling it out. The closer one sticks to the suggested mealtimes on this page, the easier it should be.

Chapter 24: Putting a Plan Together: Seek the Kingdom of Yahweh above All Things

Daily Journal

Date _____

Did I stick to my plan today?   ❏ Yes   ❏ No

Was it easy or did I have a challenge?

❏ Easy

❏ Challenge _____

What I can do to make it easier: _____

_____

_____

_____

_____

Are changes I make to my plan agreeable with Yahweh's Word?

Notes: _____

_____

_____

_____

_____

_____

CHAPTER 25

Go in Good Health:
Seek His Will, and He Will Direct Your Path!

He who farms his land will have plenty of food, but he who follows futilities has no sense. —Proverbs 12:11

Another word for health is 'energy'. You will never see a healthy person who doesn't have energy. You may see a sick person appear to have energy that may be mere stimulation. A truly healthy person is energized without the need for stimulants. Yahweh gives us the energy, but all the toxins we put in our bodies physically, emotionally, and spiritually diminish our energy levels — in essence, diminish our health.

The best way to conserve our energy and our health is to take advantage of the amazing blessings that Yahweh has in store for each and every one of us. Use His map to the treasure: the Scriptures! Science, thousands of years later, is now confirming what Yahweh told us in His Torah about what is healthiest for man. Below are four suggested steps to improve your health and receive Yahweh's blessings.

Step Number One: Eliminate the Causes of the Problem

Avoiding evil is the highway of the upright; he who watches his step preserves his life. —Proverbs 16:17

Too much stress is the most common cause of poor health. Feeling uncomfortable is stressful. All disease is really nothing but distress to the body or mind. There are many causes of stress in this world, but how we deal with these causes will determine the degree of stress we allow ourselves to reach. Today, there are many gadgets and pills to avoid getting too stressed. You don't need any of them. The best way to avoid stress is to have a close personal relationship with Yahweh.

The enemy does his best to cause people to feel overstressed. That's the only way they'll become sick — so weak in mind, body, and spirit that they will let the enemy come in and have his way with them, making their lives a living hell.

What is stressing you: guilt about overeating, your job, certain people in your life? Or is there spiritual warfare going on in your household? Change your thinking so these things don't stress you any more, or get yourself away from what it is causing so much stress in your life. Health begins with getting rid of what is causing the stress. The first step is identifying the problem so you can eliminate it.

There are many potential root causes to our sicknesses, and we must treat the true causes in our lives to get down to the root of the problem. Whatever the cause, we must take action and get it out of our lives once we identify it!

A good way to identify that you are unhealthy is to observe your digestion. People who are stressed seem to have weak digestion, and many times constipation is the result. If you're eating three meals a day, you should be going to the bathroom at least twice a day, or at least you should have one *big* bowel movement each day. Anything less would signal constipation or disease in your life.

Another good way to tell if you are unhealthy is by your energy level. Your energy should be at a high level most of the time. If it isn't, then you should be resting or sleeping more often and making any other necessary adjustments in your life. Find out what is zapping your energy. Once you heal and become energized again, make sure you use your energy wisely.

Another way to identify poor health is noticing that you are not feeling at your best emotionally or spirituality. Yahweh's plan is for us always to feel our best physically, emotionally, and spiritually. Our bodies are the best messengers to tell us if our current conditions are otherwise.

If you're following all the guidelines for a healthy lifestyle and still don't feel your best, it's a good sign you're detoxifying at a faster than comfortable rate, or you have a deficiency. Both of these are strong signs that you might have a disease. Not to worry, because as long as you are feeling the warning signs, it will be easy to identify them.

It's the people whose bodies have lost the capability to feel when something is wrong who should worry. Have you ever heard of someone who never gets sick and hasn't been to a doctor in years but one day wakes up with something like cancer? No one gets cancer or more advanced stages of disease without having the beginning stages of disease. The people who ignore it are the ones in whom it comes back worse. People ignore it because they do not feel the warning signs. Identifying the problem is a vital step in eliminating it.

Step Number Two: Clean and Rebuild.

Once we have figured out the primary cause of our illness and eliminated it, we next have to heal from the damage that we created.

There are many different ways to cleanse. We determine the best action to cleanse and heal depending on what the problem is. Emotionally, we can avoid things like television; physically, we can fast; and spiritually, we can pray. These are just some of the many ways we can cleanse and heal. The rebuilding process may require special attention to damaged areas. Once an area is healed, not much work will be needed to maintain a good state of health: just wisdom, knowledge, strength, and faith.

Step Number Three: Look at the Blood.

Because people are so toxic, they cannot truly feel the pain as soon as they should. This misleads us to believe we are fine when in fact we can be very sick. A good basic blood test and/or other blood test can reveal damage and disease a long time before we feel it. It can reveal if we have any deficiencies sooner than any other method.

It's also helpful to find a good doctor who knows how to read the results of the blood work. Many people don't realize it, but many doctors really don't understand the correct ranges on the blood test. Once you have your blood work, you can create a diet that works best for your own chemistry.

You can see clear signs when something is wrong in many cases. It won't be as easy in other cases. You'll have to pay really close attention to your body and its functions. Learn what is supposed to be happening. If it's not happening, then take it as a good sign that something is wrong, whether you feel it or not. Monitor your digestion, energy, sleeping patterns, and feelings.

Step Number Four: Consistently Build Your Relationship with Yahweh

Probably the greatest step we can take to help us get well and stay healthy is consistently working on our relationship with Yahweh. This could easily be Step One because we should use it to start each day of our lives and continuously stay focused on it. Study, pray, and meditate on the Scriptures. Avoid the daily distractions that keep you away from having time to do this. Gossip, news, junk magazines, etc. are just some of the common ways we waste our energies and precious time we could be spending with Yahweh.

One big problem is that so many people today focus on what other people might think of them or how they will look to the world. The answer is not to focus on results to show off to the world. Focus on the intentions of your heart and the love you have for the One who created you. The outcome will always be right if the focus is right, regardless of how it seems. Yahweh doesn't make mistakes. All we have to do is have the right focus and action, and our lives will always be joyful.

> *Don't worry about anything; on the contrary, make your requests known to Yahweh by prayer and petition, with thanksgiving.*
>
> *Then Yahweh's shalom, passing all understanding, will keep your hearts and minds safe in union with the Messiah Yeshua.*
> —Philippians 4:6-7

Today, we are such a sick world and getting sicker for one simple reason: people are doing what is popular today and listening to the word of man instead of listening to the Word of Yahweh.

I don't understand everything Yahweh asks us to do, but I do know that if He says it's not good for me, I believe He knows something I don't, and I take His Word over anyone else's.

Diagnosis
We are sick and need our Creator to heal us.

> *However, I will bring it health and healing; I will heal them and reveal to them peace and truth in plenty.* —Jeremiah 33:6

Prescription
Take one copy of the Scriptures, get some faith, and pray to Him every morning and evening.

Conclusion

> Many marvel that the human race have so degenerated physically, mentally, and morally. They do not understand it is the violation of Yahweh's constitution and laws and the violation of the laws of heath that have produced this sad degeneracy. The transgression of Yahweh's commandments has caused His prospering hand to be removed.

This was written in 1864 by Ellen White, but it is still true today. Man has still not learned from his destructive ways.

In my study of diet and spiritually, I find that most of our illness is a result of abusing Yahweh's blessings. He gave us food as nourishment, and we have taken it and made it a sinful pleasure by overconsuming everything we stuff into our bodies. Too much of a good thing can quickly become harmful and with diet usually does.

> *Here is what Yahweh says: "Stand at the crossroads and look; ask about the ancient paths, 'Which one is the good way?' Take it, and you will find rest for your souls."* —Jeremiah 6:16

It is our duty to know how to preserve the body in the very best condition of health, and it is a sacred duty to live up to the light Yahweh has graciously given us. Breaking any of the health rules Yahweh has given us is no different from breaking one of the Ten Commandments: we suffer the consequences for either.

Yahweh has given us a simple choice: life or death (Deuteronomy 30:10). We have got to make the right choice each time we sit down to eat! More people have gotten disease for not following Yahweh's eating guidelines than any other cause of sickness ever! We are committing suicide with the way we eat. We should be continually growing closer to Yahweh and becoming healthier physically, but we are going the other way when we eat in excess and the wrong foods.

I hear many people today say not "if I get sick," but "when I get sick." They don't even realize what they are saying. It wasn't much different for me. As long as there was a doctor and I had insurance, it didn't matter what was being put into my body. Once people get sick, their thoughts on the matter change. They don't want to deal with the pain.

It kind of reminds me of drinking. People go out with friends and innocently have a few drinks and a lot of fun, but a few drinks become more and more. Before they know it, they wake up with a hangover and promise they will never drink again. But a few days pass, and soon enough they are drinking again.

The first sin of man was not about eating some apple. It was about disobeying Yahweh. Just as Adam and Eve suffered for their disobedience, we continue to suffer for ours. However, we are given another chance to make things right with Yahweh's grace. Each day we have a chance to restore all the damage we have done, but we also have the choice to lose all we have gained (Ezekiel 33: 12-20).

> *Hear the word of the Creator, you Israelites, because the Creator has a charge to bring against you who live in the land:"There is no faithfulness, no love, no acknowledgment of Yahweh in the land.*
>
> *There is only cursing, lying and murder, stealing and adultery; they break all bounds, and bloodshed follows bloodshed.*
>
> *Because of this the land mourns, and all who live in it waste away; the beasts of the field and the birds of the air and the fish of the sea are dying.* —Hosea 4:1-3 [NIV]

In Hosea 4:1-3 above, our Creator is telling His chosen people of Israel that without faithfulness, knowledge, and obedience to His guidance, they will be in trouble. They will be filled with sadness, and their health will decline. So will all life around them.

This is the most important thing to remember and keep with you from this entire book: *Be faithful, kind, and continue to get knowledge and understanding of His Word*. Even if you don't understand His Word, stick to it. He is our Creator and wants only the best for you.

After traveling all over the world, and more in a year than most people ever travel in a lifetime, I've seen many eating patterns. All I can say is that people are truly addicted to eating more food than they need more often than they need it.

For many years, I was one of the chief offenders, but I became wise and obedient and stepped back from feeding that addiction. When you step back, it's much easier to see the full picture. However, when you are caught in the daily cycle of giving in to the addictions, it all appears as a matrix. It's almost impossible to see what's really going on. If you are blind to the fact that most people overeat, as I once was, there is a good chance you are suffering on one level or another.

I have discovered practicing temperance when eating will rid you of many of the health issues and help you achieve goals you have only dreamed about up to this point. Your goal should be to reduce the number of meals you consume, along with the amount of food in those meals, while making sure you are consuming the highest-quality food at the right times.

There was a plan designed for us long ago, and eventually everything will be in the end as it was at the beginning.

Everything I plan will come to pass. —Isaiah 46:10 [NLT]

It's not just the foods we consume, but when and how often we consume them, that will help us achieve our goals. We should eat less on the Sabbath, and put our focus more on Yahweh.

Do all to the Glory of Yahweh. Yeshua didn't die for us so we can live overeating, treating our bodies like trash and waste buckets. Each day we need to be thankful for Yeshua and treat our temples with respect. There is no denying it: eating and drinking have a direct bearing upon our spiritual advancement. We must free ourselves from the lust for food. We must break the patterns that have destroyed people for many years.

At the beginning of this book, we spoke about what we all truly desire. The rest of this book explained, based on the guideline of the Scriptures, that we can have all we desire if it is the will of Yahweh.

In summing up, this book told us how the Scriptures show us

how to fulfill our desires:

- a pain-free life (no painful disease): eating a diet according to the Torah!
- shalom (emotional peace): by living a life according to the Word of Yahweh
- having everlasting joy (continuous joy): by having the strongest faith always!

Trust in Yahweh with all your heart; do not depend on your own understanding.

Seek His will in all you do, and He will direct your paths.
—Proverbs 3:5-6 [NLT]

From prayer and study of His Word, I have not changed to my knowledge the meaning of any of the scriptural passages in this book. I have no agenda other than to guide you to good health and safety in accordance with what Yahweh asks us to do. I am not here to judge anyone. Your judgment is between you and Him. This book was created to guide you with His words.

If we look to man for salvation, we may easily be led astray, just as many people today are being misled. They are following man's laws instead of Yahweh's guide. A time is coming when we will all be judged not by our man-made laws, but by Yahweh's suggestions that were designed to last *forever*.

Just because man decided to replace Yahweh's requests with his own laws doesn't mean the guide originally given to us by Yahweh has changed. We are still accountable. Yahweh is the final judge, and He will judge us in His court on His time.

I believe that just because people have different belief systems doesn't mean they can't co-exist in harmony with respect for one another's diversity. Regardless of one's beliefs, each person is individually responsible for seeking Yahweh and walking in His ways.

I don't want to make this an issue of right or wrong, but it's important to put into practice whatever we can to please Yahweh the most and receive His blessings.

I observe people in love with individuals doing outrageous things to prove their love. We need to be in love with Yahweh, and the best way to show Him how much we love Him is to do our best is to learn His words and live by them.

He is our Creator who made us, and His Word is the truth. If your car broke down, you would open the glove compartment and look at the manual to see how to fix it. You also check that manual when you first get the car to see how to keep it in good working order. We are created by Him, and His manual for our well-being is the Scriptures.

If you're sick and a doctor tells you what to do to get better, would you do only some of the things he says and not listen to the rest because you didn't feel it was important enough? Chances are you would listen to the doctor and do everything he told you.

Well, if you were going to listen to a doctor and follow a doctor's orders, why wouldn't you do the same for Yahweh? He created you and knows your body better than any doctor ever will. There is no doctor better than Yahweh and no medicine better than prayer!

Some may wonder why there are some righteous people who live by His guide but also have disease. Instead of getting confused by this, understand an obedient person can have disease caused by situations in his life before becoming an obedient person, or he can be currently suffering from things out of his control; but for the most part, a righteous person will experience much better health than an unrighteous person. The appearance of this might not always be revealed at first, but in the long run, a person who knows he is pleasing Yahweh will have eternal joy on the inside regardless of what is going on with his body.

All we have to do is start living a life according to Yahweh's guide! After Yahweh made us, He gave us His safety instructions as a guide to help us live righteously. His guidebook is the Scriptures; when we live according to its teachings, we will experience health and happiness throughout life.

If you do suffer from disease, take personal responsibility and have amazing faith, knowing Yahweh will heal you. You must consistently focus on Yahweh's Word and stay strong in faith! This, along with action, will bring healing to you. Hallelu-Yah!

How blessed are those who reject the advice of the wicked, don't stand on the way of sinners, or sit where scoffers sit!

Their delight is in Yahweh's Torah; on His Torah they meditate day and night. —Psalms 1:1-2

For Yahweh watches over the way of the righteous, but the way of the wicked is doomed. —Psalms 1:6

If they obey and serve Him, they shall spend their days in prosperity, and their years in pleasures. —Job 36:11 [NKJV]

To His disciples Yeshua said, "Because of this I tell you, don't worry about your life — what you will eat or drink; or about your body — what you will wear.

"For life is more than food, and the body is more than clothing." —Luke 12:22-23

Seek good and not evil, that you may live; so Yahweh, Elohim of hosts will be with you, as you have spoken. —Amos 5:14 [NKJV]

I sought Yahweh, and He answered me; He rescued me from everything I feared. —Psalms 34:4

Earnestly seek the better gifts. And yet I show you a more excellent way. —1 Corinthians 12:31 [NKJV]

Here is my final conclusion: Fear Yahweh and obey His commands, for this is the duty of every person. —Ecclesiastes 12:13 [NLT]

List of Clean Meats and Unclean Meats

The list presented in this Appendix sums up Leviticus 11 and Deuteronomy 16. This summary is from *The Makers Diet* by Jordan Rubin.

There are four areas to consider: animal meat, fish, birds, and insects.

Animal Meat

- The clean animal meats are the flesh of animals having cloven or split hooves that also chew the cud (Leviticus 11:3). This includes cows, goats, sheep, oxen, deer, buffalo, and so forth. These can be eaten.
- Avoid animals that chew the cud, but do not have cloven or split hooves (Leviticus 11:4). This includes, but is not limited to, horses, camels, rats, skunks, dogs, cats, squirrels, and opossums.
- Do not eat swine (pigs). They have divided hooves, but they do not chew the cud. These are unclean animals (Leviticus 11:7-8). In fact, pigs are so unclean that Yahweh warns us not even to touch the body, meat, or carcass of a pig. The Hebrew words used to describe unclean meats can be translated as 'foul', 'polluted', and 'putrid'. The same terms were used to describe human waste and other disgusting substances.

Fish

Eat any fish with fins and scales, but avoid fish or water creatures without them (Leviticus 11:9-10). Those to avoid include smooth-skinned species, such as catfish or eel, and hard-shelled crustaceans, such as crab, lobster, or clams.

Birds

Birds that live primarily on insects, grubs, or grains are considered clean, but avoid birds or fowl that eat flesh (whether caught live or carrion). They are unclean. (See the extensive list in Leviticus 11:13-19.)

Insects

The Scriptures even describe edible and inedible insects in Leviticus 11:20-23, foods not normally consumed in North America. Unclean "swarming things," such as lizards, moles, mice, chameleons, and crocodiles are also listed in verses 20-31 as among those to be avoided.

Recipes

I have decided to include some of my favorite recipes made with uncooked fruits and vegetables. These recipes are quick and easy to make, have much nutrition, and go along with Genesis 1:29.

Nut Milks

Almond Milk Drink

2 to 3 cups almond milk

1 tablespoon green food powder (Pure Synergy)

2 teaspoons hemp powder

1 teaspoon green powder stevia

½ teaspoon maca powder

2 teaspoons chia seeds

¼ teaspoon camu powder

¼ teaspoon sea salt

6 ice cubes

Makes 2 servings

Process all ingredients in a blender or food processor until completely smooth.

Hemp Milk Drink

1 cup water

½ cup hemp seeds

1 tablespoon maca powder

2 teaspoons raw carob powder

½ teaspoon camu powder

1 tablespoon green powder stevia

Sea salt to taste

1 tablespoon green powder
1 tablespoon chia seeds
Ice cubes

Makes 2 servings

Process all of the ingredients in a blender or a food processor until completely smooth.

"Egg" Nog

No, this is nothing like the eggnog you're familiar with. It's better!

1 vanilla bean
2 cups almond milk
1 cup macadamia nuts
½ cup raw honey
1 tablespoon ground cinnamon
1 teaspoon ground nutmeg
¼ teaspoon turmeric
1 banana cut into 4 or 5 pieces

Makes about 4 cups

Slice the vanilla bean in half lengthwise with the tip of a sharp knife. Scrape the seeds from each half and place into blender. Add all of the remaining ingredients to the blender. Process until smooth.

Salads and Salad Dressings

Paul's Powerful Salad

I call this my "powerful" salad because every ingredient is a powerhouse of nutrients.

Fresh spinach leaves (as much as you like)

½ medium cucumber chopped

½ stalk celery chopped

1 avocado peeled, pitted, and chopped

½ red bell pepper cored, seeded, and chopped (optional)

1 to 2 tablespoons ground flaxseeds

Juice of 1 lemon

Makes 1 serving

Place the spinach, cucumber, celery, avocado, and red bell pepper (if desired) into a large bowl. Toss together to combine. Sprinkle with flaxseeds and lemon juice.

Herb Dressing

This tastes great over broccoli.

2 stalks fresh fennel

½ cup fresh cilantro

1 cup walnuts

½ onion

Sea salt to taste

½ cup nutritional yeast

Makes about 2 cups

Process all ingredients in a blender or food processor until completely smooth.

Caesar Dressing

½ cup almond butter

½ cup pine nuts

Juice of ½ lemon
2 cloves garlic
Salt to taste
Cayenne to taste

Makes about 1 cup.

Process all ingredients in a blender or food processor until completely smooth.

Red Tahini

½ cup sesame seeds
2 cloves garlic
Juice from ½ lemon
½ red bell pepper
Cayenne to taste

Makes about 1 cup

Process all ingredients in a blender or food processor until completely smooth.

Carrot Ginger Salad Dressing

5 carrots
2-inch piece fresh ginger
¼ cup water or apple cider vinegar
1 date

Makes about 2 cups

Process all ingredients in a blender or food processor until completely smooth.

Sesame Ginger Dressing

¼ cup fresh lemon juice
1½ inch piece fresh ginger peeled
¼ cup raw sesame oil or olive oil
1 large clove garlic
1 teaspoon kelp powder
Pinch cayenne

Makes about ½ cup

Process all ingredients into a blender or food processor until completely smooth.

Almond Ginger Dressing

2 cups chopped bell pepper
1 cup raw almond butter
½ cup chopped scallion
¼ cup chopped red beet
2 teaspoons chopped fresh ginger
1 clove garlic
1½ teaspoons kelp powder
1 cup water
1 tablespoon nama shoyu
½ tablespoon fresh lemon juice
Cayenne to taste

Makes about 4 cups

Process all ingredients in a blender or food processor until completely smooth.

Cheddar Sauce

1 cup raw cashews, sunflower seeds, or almonds
½ large red bell pepper
¼ cup water
2 tablespoons fresh lemon juice
2 tablespoons nutritional yeast
1 tablespoon tahini
1½ teaspoons sea salt
1 clove garlic
2 teaspoons onion power, 1 small slice onion, or 1 tablespoon chopped green onion.

Makes about 2 cups

Process all ingredients in a blender or food processor until completely smooth, adding the water a little at a time until it reaches desired consistency.

Tomato Basil Dressing

This dressing is especially delicious in late summer when you're assured of fresh, ripe tomatoes and basil.

2 tomatoes cut into quarters
1 clove garlic
Juice of ½ medium lemon
1 cup fresh basil leaves

Makes about 2 cups

Process all ingredients into a blender or food processor until completely smooth.

Dips, Spreads, and Sauces

Raw, Healthful Pesto

Serve as a dip or over pasta.

>2 to 4 cloves garlic
>2 bunches spinach
>1 bunch fresh basil
>Juice of ½ medium lemon
>1 cup pine nuts
>½ teaspoon Celtic sea salt
>½ cup olive oil
>
>Makes 4 servings

Place garlic into a food processor. Process until the garlic is well minced. Add all remaining ingredients and process until completely smooth.

Tomato Sauce

I also like to add a chopped avocado to this and serve it with raw pasta dishes.

>3 tomatoes
>½ cup sundried tomatoes (not packed in oil)
>1 clove garlic
>½ tablespoon chopped fresh basil
>½ tablespoon chopped fresh oregano
>1 small hot pepper, such as a jalapeño or serrano
>
>Makes about 2 cups

Place all ingredients into a blender or food processor. Process until completely smooth.

Pine Nut Dip

Pour this over a raw salad, or use it as a dip for fresh, raw vegetables.

1 cup pine nuts
½ lemon
¼ teaspoon ground nutmeg
1-inch piece fresh ginger peeled
1 clove garlic
Sea salt to taste

Makes 2 cups

Place all ingredients into a blender or food processor. Process until well combined.

Onion-Walnut Pâté

This is great served with raw vegetables, or serve sliced as an entrée.

1 cup minced onion
¼ cup loosely packed parsley
2 cups soaked walnuts
2 teaspoons pine nuts
Sea salt to taste

Makes 5 to 8 servings

Process all ingredients into a blender or food processor until completely smooth.

Chia Tapioca Pudding

¼ cup chia seeds
1 cup almond, banana, or coconut milk

2 tablespoons raw raisins

Ground cinnamon to taste

Makes about 1½ cups

In a medium bowl, mix chia seeds and milk. Place into refrigerator for 10 minutes. Add raisins and stir in cinnamon. Return to refrigerator overnight, stirring several times. You may need to stir once again before serving.

Blended Meals

Blended Salad

For better digestion, try drinking your salads instead of chewing them. Here's one of my favorites:

1 cup spinach or lettuce leaves

½ medium cucumber cut into 3 or 4 pieces

1 stalk celery cut into 3 or 4 pieces

Juice of ½ lemon

1 avocado pitted and peeled

1 tomato roughly chopped

1 cup sunflower sprouts (optional)

½ red bell pepper cored, seeded, and cut into 4 or 5 pieces (optional)

1 teaspoon flaxseed or olive oil (optional)

Makes 2 to 3 servings

Process all ingredients into a blender or food processor until completely smooth.

Coconut Avocado Drink

Coconut and avocado make a surprisingly good combination.

>Meat and water from 1 young coconut
>1 avocado pitted and peeled

>Makes 1 serving

Process all ingredients into a blender or food processor until completely smooth.

Coconut, Spinach, and Avocado Drink

Spinach gives this unusual drink more depth of flavor.

>Meat and water from 1 young coconut
>1 cup spinach leaves or other greens
>1 avocado pitted and peeled

>Makes 2 cups

Place the coconut meat and water into a blender. Process until smooth. Add the spinach and avocado. Process again until smooth.

Resources

PAUL NISON
P.O. Box 16156
West Palm Beach, FL 33416
Toll-free 866-729-7285, or 866-RAW-PAUL
E-mail: paul@rawlife.com
www.paulnison.com

This is the official website of author and raw food chef Paul Nison. See the website for Paul's teaching and lecture schedule.

RAW LIFE, INC.
P.O. Box 16156
West Palm Beach, FL 33416
Toll-free 866-729-7285, or 866-RAW-PAUL
E-mail: paul@rawlife.com
www.rawlife.com

This is the best website for health books on all topics, including raw food diets and spiritual health. It also has a good selection of the highest-quality raw food health snacks, foods, and supplements.

TORAH LIFE MINISTRIES
P.O. Box 16156
West Palm Beach, FL 33416
Toll-free 866-729-7285, or 917-407-2270
E-mail: paul@rawlife.com
www.torahlifeministries.org

Torah Life Ministries, Inc. is a nonprofit ministry teaching the Word of Yahweh, proclaiming the Good News of Yeshua, and supporting the healing of all by revealing a more excellent way.

It is in our hearts to help fellow believers understand the important health message found in the Scriptures without having to deal with all the "New Age" stuff associated with so many health teachings today!

We are also here to

- Strengthen families worldwide
- Teach the Hebrew roots of the faith
- Expose pagan practices of religion
- Experience true worship

To contact us and for donations, address all correspondence and donations to:

Torah Life Ministries
P.O. Box 16156
West Palm Beach, FL 33416
Toll-free 866-729-7285, or 866-RAW-PAUL
Email: paul@rawlife.com

Please make checks out to Torah Life Ministries.

About the Author

At age 20, Paul Nison was diagnosed with inflammatory bowel disease (also known as Crohn's disease and ulcerative colitis), a deadly affliction.

His search for a cure began with medical doctors, but they didn't have the answers he needed. After trying almost every so-called cure to overcome his pain and suffering, Paul finally discovered the benefits of eating more simply. He started by getting rid of foods that were no good for him. Simplifying his diet was the first step in his cure.

"I was eating so much unhealthful food but didn't care because I felt great. When I got very sick, I finally realized health doesn't start with what we add to our diet, but with what we leave out."

Paul started to eliminate all unhealthful foods. The healthful foods he was left with were raw, ripe, fresh, organic fruits, vegetables, nuts, and seeds.

After turning to a simpler diet known as the raw food diet, consisting of just that, raw foods, Paul became amazed at how quickly his health returned. He was even more amazed because doctors had told him raw foods would not help his condition. In fact, they warned him against it by saying that a diet of raw fruits and vegetables would be harmful to anyone with inflammatory bowel disease.

This led Paul to simplify all areas of his life. With his new understanding of "less is more," Paul left his office job in the financial industry on Wall Street in New York City, wrote some books about health, and started traveling, giving lectures about health and living simply.

Paul didn't know it at the time, but his return to health and a simpler lifestyle was just the beginning of a path that would bring him to question the connection between today's fast-paced urban lifestyle and the sadly diseased state in which so many people find themselves. "The more I started to realize what was really going on, the more I would see most people moving around like robots, barely surviving, while I was thriving."

This led Paul to continue to search for an answer. He realized that people are being controlled by the world. Most of the people in control do not have the best interests of the people they are controlling at heart.

As Paul continued to study, he was led to read the Bible. When he saw that it clearly said we should not be controlled by the people of the world, but by the Master Creator, Father Yahweh, everything made perfect sense.

As definitive confirmation that our Creator and not the world had all the answers, Paul found Genesis 1:29:

> *See, I have given you every plant that yields seed which is on the face of all the earth, in which there is life, every green plant is for food.*

"Discovering healthful eating was a big step for me, but finally building a personal relationship with our Creator was the biggest. My life has definitely changed. It is better than it ever was."

Paul's life is now dedicated to studying and living according to the Scriptures and to developing his relationship with the Most High. It is Paul's prayer to help as many people as possible see the amazing health message of the Scriptures and to help them get to know and understand their Creator. According to Paul, the Scriptures comprise the greatest book on health ever written.

To convey his message, Paul will travel wherever he must. He spends much of his time on the road. Paul explains that the hectic life on the road working many hours is only possible with the help of Our Creator.

"There is so much to get done, but each second I spend working on this is a joy because I know it's not for me; it is for our Creator, and it is helping people."

Paul usually speaks at health food stores, retreats, churches, Messianic assemblies, yoga studios, parks, and corporate offices.

Paul says there is nowhere he wouldn't speak, as long as people are interested in helping themselves get better.

Paul is on a mission to bring the message of health and healing to the world. His experiences and background in raw food nutrition, along with his study of the Scriptures, have helped him develop a unique teaching style that is fun, simple, and to the point. Paul has helped people in several countries achieve their goals while pleasing their Maker.

He's known among his peers as a humble and enjoyable person to be around, while he speaks boldly and to the point at the same time. He has a unique style, combining humor and boldness to get his message across to everyone. From children to seniors, men and women, everyone stands to benefit from Paul's message.

Suggested Reading

Health Books
Books by Paul Nison

Healing Inflammatory Bowel Disease: The Cause and Cure of Crohn's Disease and Ulcerative Colitis

Raw Knowledge: Enhancing the Powers of The Mind, Body and Soul

The Daylight Diet: Divine Eating for Superior Health and Digestion

Paul Nison's Raw Food Formula for Health: A Modern Approach to Health through Simplicity, Variety and Moderation

The Raw Life: Becoming Natural in an Unnatural World

Books by Other Authors

Become Younger by Dr. Norman Walker

Fit for Life by Harvey and Marilyn Diamond

God's Key to Health and Happiness by Elmer A. Josephson

How We All Went Raw: Raw Food Recipe Book by Charles Nungesser and Stephen Malachi

Living Foods for Optimum Health by Brian Clement

Rational Fasting by Arnold Ehret

The Cause and Cure of All Human Illness by Arnold Ehret

The Entering Wedge, published by Victor T. Houteff

The Healing Oils of the Bible by Jim Lynn

The Hippocrates Diet by Ann Wigmore

The Maker's Diet by Jordan S. Rubin

The Miracle of Fasting by Paul Bragg

The Mucusless Diet Healing System by Arnold Ehret

Essential Daily Reading

The most recommended book of all: The Scriptures of our Creator!

Prayers

You can change your health and your life for the better right now, just as I did. You can pray right now where you are.

Prayer to Repent

"Father Yahweh, give me the wisdom and understanding to know your will for my life. Please heal sickness and disease from my body. Strengthen me to persevere over temptation when my flesh is weak. I need your words to guide me, your spirit to help me, and your Son Yeshua in my heart. I pray Father that Your will be done in my life, and I will continually seek your guidance. I pray all these things in your Son Yeshua's name."

Prayer to Change Your Life

"Father Yahweh, I know that I have made mistakes in my life, and I ask for your forgiveness. I believe that Yeshua, the Messiah, died for my sins and rose from the dead. I invite you into my life to be my Elohim and my Savior. I ask you to come into my life and make me a part of your family forever."

If you sincerely put your faith in Yeshua, the Messiah, our Creator promises not only to forgive you, but also to receive you into His family.

This is the greatest discovery you will ever make!

❏ I have just prayed to receive Yeshua into my life. Please send me free literature to help me grow in my new relationship with my Maker, Yahweh.

Name:	_____
Age: _____ **Date:**	_____
Address:	_____
City: _____ **State:** _____ **Zip:**	_____
Country:	_____
Email Address:	_____
Phone Number:	_____

Please copy or cut out this form, and mail with check, money order, or bank draft payable in US currency to:

Paul Nison • P.O. Box 16156 • West Palm Beach, FL 33416

As time goes by, the mailing address may change several times. Please check www.paulnison.com, or call for the most updated contact information.

To contact the author for speaking engagements, call toll free 866-RAW-PAUL (866-729-7285) or e-mail paul@rawlife.com.

Index

A

Abraham
12, 139, 196, 210

animal products
62, 66, 84, 96, 227

animals
27, 30, 59, 64-70, 73-84, 87, 95, 106-107, 112, 137, 147, 151, 197, 227, 243

appointed
40, 58, 107, 127, 132, 140, 151, 185

B

Bible
xi, xv, xvii-xxvii, 63, 67, 75, 80, 88, 102, 158, 175, 258, 262

blood
xxi, xxviii, 6, 61, 66-69, 71, 73, 76, 79-81, 90, 100-101, 104, 106, 109, 151, 202, 217, 219, 233, 267

C

cheese
5, 78-79, 105

chlorophyll
99-102

clean meats
106, 243

D

detoxification
ii, 123, 215, 226

diet
ii, ix-x, xv, xvii-xxiii, xxv, 3-8, 21-25, 34-35, 38, 44, 51, 53-55, 62-66, 68-70, 73, 79-80, 83-85, 88, 90, 95-96, 100, 102-103, 106, 109, 111, 119, 126-127, 131, 136, 140-141, 143, 155-156, 159-160, 182-183, 198-199, 214, 218, 220, 223-227, 233, 237, 240, 243, 257, 261, 262, 269

digestion
53, 89, 102, 118, 121, 123-126, 134, 144, 149, 152, 157, 232, 234, 253, 261, 269

disease
x-xi, xvii-xviii, xix-xxii, 3, 6, 9, 14, 16-17, 19, 21, 22, 25-28, 31, 34, 37, 39-40, 42-43, 46, 59-60, 63, 74, 81, 88, 101, 103, 110, 114, 119-121, 123, 131, 159, 163, 168, 173-174, 179-180, 184-185, 191-199, 201-202, 209-211, 216, 219, 224, 231-233, 237, 240-241, 257, 261, 263, 267, 269

doctors
xvii-xviii, 6-7, 18, 35, 62, 81, 202, 209-210, 233, 257

F

fasting
158-159, 168, 225-226, 261-262

fresh
4, 7, 35, 55, 57, 59, 62, 78, 90, 96-97, 99, 141, 159, 227, 247-252, 257

G

Garden of Eden
14, 55, 60, 66, 95, 118

gas
126

goat
105-107

god
xi, xvii, xix, xxvii, 82, 144, 167, 261

good news
18, 63, 184, 202, 210, 214, 255, 267

grains
76, 86, 88-89, 105, 244

grape juice
89-91

grass
78, 84, 102, 106, 205

H

Hallelu-Yah
xvi, 10, 14-15, 19-21, 23, 209, 242

healing
xi, xiii, xvii, xix, xxiii, 3, 9-10, 15, 18, 31, 59-60, 84, 89, 123, 134-135, 156, 158-159, 168, 179, 186, 193-194, 201-202, 204-207, 209-210, 213-214, 216, 235, 242, 255, 258, 261-262, 267, 269

Hebrew
iii, xxvii, 26, 31, 38, 75, 243, 255

Hebrews
16, 37, 67, 75, 170, 192

Holy Spirit
xxvii, 14

I

Isaac
12

Israel
13, 27, 38, 77, 80, 95, 152, 197, 238

J

Jacob
12, 139

Jesus
ix, xxi, xxvii

Jewish
xxvii, 13, 38, 70, 112, 126, 151

Job
45, 118, 120, 172, 178, 242

joy
i, xx-xxi, xxiii, 3, 10, 14, 18-19, 22, 29-32, 41, 45, 48, 171, 173, 184, 197, 206, 240-241, 258, 269

juice
4-5, 7, 89-91, 159, 226, 247-251, 253

K

knowledge
iv, xi, xiii-xxii, 9, 18, 20, 23, 27-28, 40, 45-49, 53, 56-58, 60, 64-65, 77, 85, 92, 118, 144, 179-181, 197, 199, 202, 204, 206, 217, 223, 225, 233, 238, 240, 261, 267

kosher
80

L

laziness
9, 119, 138

lazy
53, 138, 163, 201

live foods
98

Lord
xix, xxvii

M

milk
7, 66, 78-79, 105-106, 245-246, 252-253

minerals
61, 84, 96, 98, 102-104

Moses
ix, 20, 37, 40, 42, 56, 68, 71, 139, 169-170, 172, 192

N

Noah
40-41, 67-68, 70, 170-172, 174-176

nuts
xvii, 7, 62, 70, 78, 98, 102, 182, 246-247, 251-252, 257

O

organic
7, 35, 78, 84, 86-88, 96-97, 104, 106, 227, 257

oxygen
81, 100-101

P

pain
8, 10, 18, 31, 180, 195, 199, 201, 224, 233, 238, 240, 257

Passover
69, 81, 140

prayer
xix, xxiii, 8, 40-41, 43, 113, 156, 168, 184, 193, 202, 204-210, 212, 217, 234, 240-241, 258, 263

R

raw
xv, xvii, 7, 35, 78-79, 96, 98, 103-106, 126, 182, 218, 220, 227, 245-246, 249-253, 255, 257-258, 261, 269

ripe
97

S

Sabbath
117, 127-128, 140-141, 145, 158, 239

saints
131

scriptures
i, iv, ix-xi, xiii-xiv, xvii-xx, xxii-xxiv, xxviii, 8-19, 21-23, 26-27, 30-31, 37-42, 45, 47-49, 51, 55-56, 58-60, 62-64, 68-71, 74-84, 88-89, 100, 105-109, 111, 114, 117-118, 120-121, 127-128, 131-132, 136-137, 140, 143-144, 151-152, 158, 162-164, 167-169, 173-174, 177, 179, 181, 186-187, 189, 195-197, 201, 203, 205-207, 209, 213, 218, 223-224, 231, 234-235, 239, 241, 244, 255, 258, 262, 269

sea vegetables
101, 103-105

seeds
102

Set-apart Spirit
xxvii, 14, 16, 23, 29, 58, 89, 201, 206

Shabbat
128

sickness
iv, xx, 16, 19, 21, 28, 31, 38, 46-47, 74, 114, 120, 136, 148, 173-174, 191-192, 194, 196, 199, 202-204, 210-212, 219, 224, 237, 263, 267

soil
84-85, 97-98, 103-104, 109, 171

sugar
62, 86-88, 90, 101, 104, 106, 142, 217, 225-227

supplements
109, 110, 255

T

Testament
11-12, 38, 56

Torah
iii, x, xx-xxi, xxiv, xxviii, 15, 17, 26, 30, 37-38, 41-42, 48, 53-57, 65, 67-69, 75,

95, 101, 107, 111, 114, 118, 128, 152, 167-168, 169, 171-172, 174-175, 177-178, 181, 186, 191, 198, 206, 224-225, 231, 240, 242, 255-256, 267, 269

V

vegan
7, 66, 70, 85, 95-96, 103, 182

vegetables
xvii, 7, 60-62, 66, 70, 77-78, 82, 84, 86, 95-96, 98-105, 220, 227, 245, 252, 257

W

water
12, 55, 79, 81, 89, 97, 99, 103, 107, 136, 145, 148, 174, 205, 216, 226, 228, 243, 245, 248-250, 254

wild
77, 79, 98-99, 112, 175, 205

wine
88-93, 178

Y

Yahweh
x, xiii-xiv, xvi, xix-xxv, xxvii, xxviii, 8-23, 25-33, 35, 38-48, 53-90, 92, 95-96, 101-102, 106-107, 109, 112-115, 117, 119-120, 122-125, 127-128, 131-141, 143-146, 148, 151-153, 155-160, 162-164, 167-179, 181, 184-187, 191-199, 201- 214, 217-218, 220, 223-225, 229, 231-232, 234, 237-243, 255, 258, 263-264, 267

Yeshua
xvi, xxi-xxiii, xxv, xxvii-xxviii, 9, 12, 14-19, 29-30, 35-37, 47-48, 54, 56-58, 62, 67-69, 71, 76, 79-80, 83, 85, 89-90, 100, 106, 111-112, 114, 143, 145, 152, 169, 172, 174-177, 184-187, 194, 198, 201-203, 206-208, 210, 234, 239, 242, 255, 263-264, 267

Torah Life Ministries

For the Son of Man did not come to destroy men's lives but to save them. —Luke 9:56 [NKJV]

There were foolish people who suffered affliction because of their crimes and sins;

they couldn't stand to eat anything; they were near the gates of death.

In their trouble they cried to Yahweh, and He rescued them from their distress;

He sent his word and healed them, He delivered them from destruction. —Psalms 107:17-20

Yeshua Heals

Yeshua went about all the towns and villages, teaching in their synagogues, proclaiming the Good News of the Kingdom, and healing every kind of disease and weakness. —Matthew 9:35

Yahweh	Yeshua
Saves — from Sin	Teaches — knowledge that will save us
Heals — from Sickness	Preaches — the good news to heal us
Delivers — from Satan	Heals — by His redeeming blood

Order Form

Item Description	Cost	Number of Copies	Total Cost
Healing Inflammatory Bowel Disease: The Cause and Cure of Crohn's Disease and Ulcerative Colitis	Book - US $11.99 per copy		
Paul Nison's Raw Food Formula for Health: A Modern Approach to Health Through Simplicity, Variety, and Moderation	Book - US $12.95 per copy		
	DVD - US $19.95 per video.		
The Daylight Diet: Divine Eating for Superior Health and Digestion	Book - US $24.95 per copy		
	DVD - US $19.95 per video		
	CD - US $9.95 per audio		
Health according to the Scriptures: Experience the Joy of Health according to Our Creator	Book - US $19.95 per copy		
	DVD - US $19.95 per video		
	CD - US $9.95 per audio		

US Shipping and Handling: $3.50 per first item, $1.00 for each additional item.

Outside the United States: $10.00 per first item, $6.00 for each additional item

Subtotal	
Shipping	
Total Amount Enclosed	

Ship to: (Please Print)

Name: _____

Address: _____

_____

City: _____ State: _____ Zip: _____

Country: _____

Email Address: _____

Phone Number: _____

Please copy or cut out this form, and mail with check, money order, or bank draft payable in US currency to:

Paul Nison • P.O. Box 16156 • West Palm Beach, FL 33416

Please make all checks payable to Raw Life. Donation to Torah Life Ministries.

As time goes by, the mailing address may change several times. Please check www.paulnison.com, or call for the most updated contact information.

To contact the author for speaking engagements, call toll free 866-RAW-PAUL (866-729-7285) or e-mail paul@rawlife.com.

Dear friend, I am praying that everything prosper with you and that you be in good health, as I know you are prospering spiritually.
—3 John 1:2.